HEALING THE FUTURE

...the triumph of spirit over flesh, choice over drift...

Healing (literally, *to make whole*) is to *no disease* as a computer is to a typewriter. This book is about the forgotten art and science of healing: an attempted tip off on the little secrets of holistic living that can be mastered in easy, small steps. Equally, it is an attempt at interpreting the ancient *Upanishadic* wisdom through the prism of the author's own experiences: to help place your evolving destiny in your own deft hands. As you take time off to muse on the alphabet of healing, make no mistake: you have begun *'the journey within'*.

Healing the Future

The Journey Within

Deepak Kashyap

New Age Books

ISBN: 81-7822-039-3

Second Revised Edition: Delhi, 2003

First Edition: Delhi, 2001

Published by

NEW AGE BOOKS

A-44 Naraina Phase-I

New Delhi-110 028 (INDIA)

Email: nab@vsnl.in

Website: www.newagebooksindia.com

Printed in India

at Shri Jainendra Press

A-45 Naraina Phase-I, New Delhi-110 028

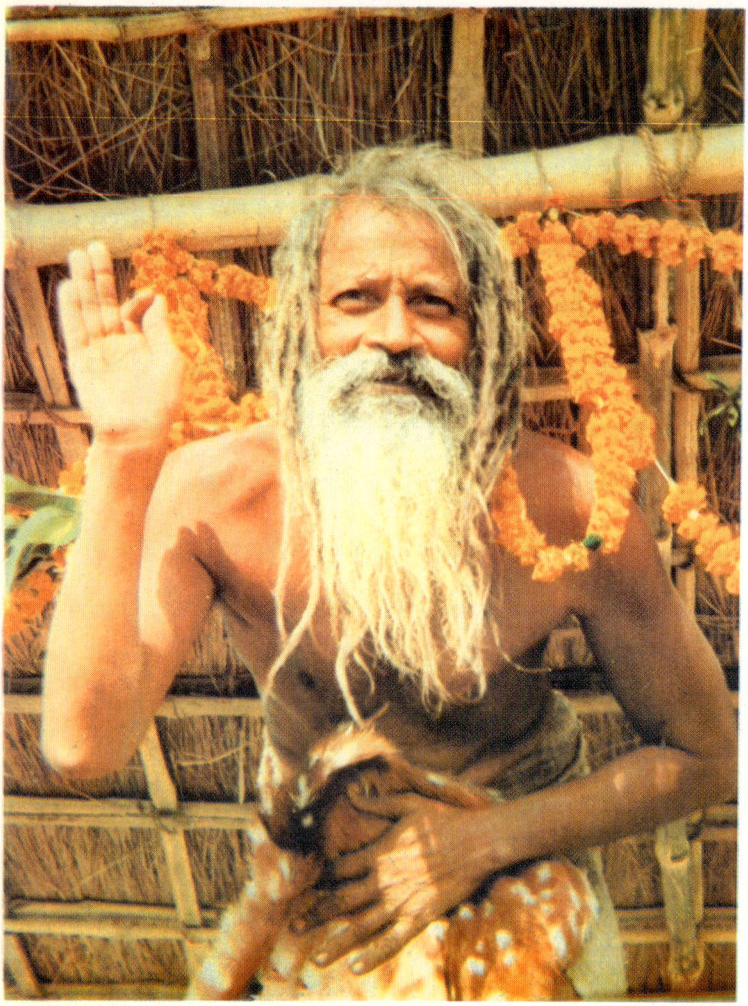

YOGI HANS BABA

Dedicated to my Siddha Guru,
*Paramahansa Devraha Hans Baba**
whose divine fire now consumes and
nourishes me every moment.

* Described by K.N. Rao as among the greatest yogis of Patanjali tradition ever seen in the plains by mankind.

Acknowledgements

This book wouldn't have been possible but for a myriad extra-ordinary influences on my life. In deciphering some of them, I am led to:

- Swami Muktananda Paramahansa whose scriptural teachings have been the greatest intellectual influence on me ever since I turned to Yoga.
- Paramahansa Yogananda whose inspired narratives were always a source of strength in my moments of indecisiveness.
- My parents, Late Sri Bhola Nath and Satya Devi, and wife Madhulika who gave me priceless emotional support during my difficult years of transition.
- Sri K.N. Rao for his amazing spiritual and astrological insights of which I have been a direct and indebted beneficiary.
- Fritjof Capra, author of *'The Tao of Physics'*, and his keynote address at the Los Angeles Symposium in 1977.
- Georg Feuerstein, whose *'The Shambhala Encyclopedia of Yoga'* helped me bring technical details of yoga theory to the reader in easy-to-understand language.

New Delhi
19-05-2001

DEEPAK KASHYAP
(deepakkashyap02@yahoo.com)

Contents

Preface to the Second Edition

Just a few Words.....

1. The key to success in yoga is in trying not too hard; in cumulatively investing more in life than you take from it. Considering that yoga is more about attitude than effort, it should reflect in everything you do. Launching of this book therefore, had to be of a piece with its writing: unostentatious and without hype.
2. Yet the response has been overwhelming. Quantitatively, it has meant the book going into this second edition in just about a year. Qualitatively, it reflects in the messages pouring in from readers all over who could lay their hands on the book in the short time.
3. Writers, asked how they came up with their most memorable works, love to say things like "the book wrote itself". Much as I would prefer avoiding the cliché, there is no denying that true creativity oozes from a state of awareness that, fleetingly, blurs all 'I'ness and captures the Infinite. In hindsight, I would like to believe that this book was equally a product of reason and the result of ecstasy. For, more than anything else, it was an attempt to fuse commonsense, science and spirituality into an organic whole. Indeed, today as never before, the physicist smashing the atom in his bubble chamber, the biologist grappling with the DNA code, the surgeon exploring pseudo-surgery as a powerful therapeutic tool, and the yogi silently meditating in a snowy Himalayan cave, are all using vastly different methods to arrive at the same inescapable conclusion. That Reality - call it the self, call it universe - is one seamless, endless, animate whole. What better way to grasp it than by taking it head on! So take the plunge if you are game.

4. Predictably, there have been a few angry reactions from well-meaning reiki-enthusiasts who just can't see how practicing this ancient healing art could conceivably boomerang. Reiki has become a big money-spinner now: something of an industry. At the risk of being politically incorrect nonetheless, I would reiterate that the present-day reiki 'experts', not to talk of the reiki-practitioners at large, are either themselves blind to its full karmic import, or don't want people to see it for reasons more commercial than spiritual.
5. A lot of curiosity seems to have been generated in Paramahansa Devraha Hans Baba—my Siddha Guru—after the book has carried a chapter on him. His inscrutable 'cosmic agenda' seems to be unfinished as yet if the relentless roaming about of this Himalayan yogi in cities of north and eastern India is any indication. Last winter, he was in Delhi. For the first time in all these years, I saw him—bare-bodied as usual—giving off just a hint of uneasiness: coughing occasionally in the biting Delhi cold. And for a change, this time he was explicit: it "came quick" from a suffering female-disciple of his sitting at 20 yards, 'leaving her to enter him just as he eyed her'. Baba, affectionate as ever, said he would now have to "throw out the damn thing fast; away from the crowd". So much for spiritual healing!
6. If I were to leave aside the grace of God Almighty and my Guru which has quite obviously been behind the relative success of my this endeavour, I have to once again deeply acknowledge the contribution of Mr. K.N. Rao who, selflessly, took maximum interest in the book and its fortunes. His formally releasing the book from the Bharatiya Vidya Bhavan premises, and now his willingness to list my book at his own website, is something I value greatly. To me, his showing so much interest in my work is as much a reflection of its inherent worth as of his own noble spirit.
7. In the tenth and concluding chapter of the book, under the sub-head 'Nature Care', I had written: "*For some cosmic reason, these natural and man-made disasters are greatly*

on the rise of late. Reliable Vedic astrologers, specially K.N. Rao, foresee the period 1999 to 2002 as particularly difficult for humanity at large....". This was well before black 11 September and its aftermath. From my meetings with yogis and genuine astrologers, I know it for a fact that much more is still to come before things start improving: hopefully after 2002. But I also tentatively realize that the fury of the holocaust can be significantly abated if mankind tilted more towards the yoga way of life and collectively made use of the soul-force for 'global health'. Is America listening?

New Delhi,
10.09.2002

Deepak Kashyap
(deepakkashyap02@yahoo.com)

Preface

From the late teens, I have been fascinated no end by the occult and the hereafter even though I was always loathe to being religious in the generally accepted sense of the term. The great hiatus between the haves and the have-nots, the apparent dysfunctioning of the much vaunted doctrine of karma and the generally evident rupturing of the social and moral order, all largely in the Indian/Subcontinental context, appeared to be reason enough not to fancy the chances of the existence of God, in whatever form. Indeed, the problem of evil has been the thorniest one in the path of theists and philosophers down the ages—"if God is Good, He cannot be Omnipotent and vice versa." I carried this "intellectually correct" notion of God and godmen for most of my early adulthood. Often, I earned the wrath of friends and familymen for calling the mushrooming roadside temples traffic hazards and for deriding pundits as social vermins. Inquisitive though I was, there was no way I could be coerced into believing in anything 'beyond and after' through a *sadhu's* sleight of the hand or a theologist's woolly discourses. Then, through a quirk of fate and bang in the middle of what should have been the most rewarding phase of my burgeoning career, I plunged into the darkest recesses of my life; forcing me to deeply introspect and recharter my life at this rather late stage in a desperate bid to 'make something click'. The more I tried to come out of the quagmire, the deeper I sank till a stage was reached when my analytical mind, my foresight and the will to fight, all appeared to have deserted me. It was at this juncture that I, the 'rationalist' cried for divine help and in fact tentatively dabbled in the occult. What followed thereafter was an amazing roller-coaster 'journey back' in mysticism that at times literally, left me gasping for breath. Over the years, this budding romance with the paranormal now seems to have made way for a more mature co-existence with a fascinating world of Yoga that has the 'miraculous' or the 'supernormal' entwined with it at each step. Ever since, I started feeling sort of duty-bound to share my rather fortuitous, yet invaluable insights into a completely higher way of living that was healing and vivifying beyond imagination, and that was yet open to all those who cared to listen. In this strange and shadowy world of seers that had tantalizingly part-opened on me to show glimpses of the unknown dimensions of human existence, my mental state was not unlike that of the diminutive Gulliver in the land of giants who lived to tell his tale to fellowmen. With this difference that in my case, I was the Gulliver and I had to be my Jonathan Swift !

It is in the above background that I started toying with the idea of writing about the science and art of practical spiritualism as I have understood. What made me dither was essentially a reluctance to join the bandwagon, as I have always held the yoga way of life to be a very scientific, yet sacred subject. To me it was a subject, not to be trifled with without the requisite preparedness, as was the case with most New Age writings on the subject. My ambivalence was after all, not without a basis. I would start with the cons first. In this age of dot coms and ' instant karma', there appears to be no dearth of literature on this subject. The new-found wisdom on meditation and yoga, through a process of reverse osmosis as it were, has travelled from the West to the Orient in such deluge and frenzy that adding to the bulk appeared to be nothing short of a crime. On the other hand, having gone through so much of available reading and practising material on the subject, I came to the uneasy realisation that by and large yoga/meditation was being presented to the layman in either of the two ways: (a) by the revivalists in a classical form that, though well meaning, was too esoteric, convoluted and even scary for the ordinary mortal; or worse, (b) by a set of unscrupulous elements who knew nothing of Yoga, but were peddling meditation, mantra and allied concepts in a ready-to-serve package that was hollow in substance and deceitful in intent. The average yoga enthusiast has therefore got put off by the rigours of the "real stuff," and often on the rebound, been claimed by the 'market forces' with their alluring promise of fixing the mind, body and soul in one go, for a fortune of course.

Particularly unfortunate has been the tendency among the yoga-conscious to become more and more physically inclined—aiming for more and more complex bodily postures and breathing techniques—in a misconceived zeal to get the yoga practice rid of its etheric or 'unscientific' component. In modern physics as well as yoga scriptures, energy is seen as the fundamental nature of existence. In the ultimate analysis, there is no solid matter. The human anatomy, our thoughts and emotions are all composed of energy vibrating at various frequencies. The kinkier the vibration, the more likely we are to experience stress or disease. The finer the vibration, the greater the chance for physical and mental well-being. New Age science is therefore, in perfect agreement with the teachings of the perfected yogis (*Siddhas*) as well as with some of my own experiences, that the richest and quickest bounties of yoga, even from a purely utilitarian point of view, can be accessed by proceeding from the mind side in the mind-body continuum. Simply put, the mind shapes the body much more than the body shapes the mind. The yoga beginners therefore, would do themselves a world of good by consciously starting to think of themselves as energy vibrations rather than solid matter. As for myself, I do recognize the place of the *hatha-yoga* component in the overall scheme of things and have often successfully overcome minor ailments through specific *asanas*. I have nonetheless seen a combination of simpler, more 'energy oriented' techniques of mind-management pay wonderful dividends even in the near-total absence of *hatha-yoga* practices. Likewise, the unsuspecting converts to the contrived New Age techniques of breathing need to be firmly told that yogic breathing happens on its own when the seeker's psyche and physique are up to it. When one practises advanced meditation, *Kevala Kumbhaka* or natural retention of breath without *Puraka* (inhalation) and *Rechaka* (exhalation) comes by itself; when *Kevala Kumbhaka* comes, one enjoys immense peace and exhilaration. That the conscious practice of *pranayama* in today's fast life is a double-edged weapon ought to be hammered into the minds of the New Age yoga-enthusiast before it is too late. Sample this: the *Gheranda-Samhita*, one of the most authentic manuals on *hatha-yoga,* lists four essential prerequisites for *pranayama*-practice—(a) *sthana*, or right place, (b) *kala*, or right time, (c) *mitahara*, or controlled diet and (d) *nadi-shuddhi*, or purification of the psycho-energetic channels that carry the life force or *prana*. The *Hatha-Yoga-Pradipika*, another medieval classic on *hatha-yoga*, cautions: "*Just as a lion, an elephant or a tiger is tamed gradually, so should the life force (through pranayama) be controlled; lest it kills the practitioner*." And the *Shiva-Samhita* forbids *pranayama*-practice shortly after a meal or when hungry.

When I saw some of the most Westernized people viewing and practising yoga in terms of some isolated physical exercises and breathing techniques unmindful of its necessary spiritual underpinnings, I felt somewhat like a computer-buff who would grow impatient with an upstart inclined to use the personal computer exclusively as a typewriter. Yes, the PC can type and type beautifully. But it can do much more; it can edit, it can instruct, it can play chess, and it can do a whole lot of things, even connect you to the Super Computer. Similarly, I now knew and wanted to tell any one who cared to listen that yoga could bring you relaxation, good health and mental peace; but it could—and was meant to—do a lot more; even connect one to God or the Supreme

Intelligence. In the event I clearly saw the need and space for a detailed exposition on yoga that combined the authenticity of the teachings of the orthodox school with the simplicity and directness of the trendy meditation packages now flooding the market. In an age of vulgar consumerism when peace, bliss and even *nirvana* have become saleable commodities, the ultimate objective of any meaningful initiative in this direction, could be only one, viz., presenting yoga and meditation to the average yoga enthusiast in such honest, uncomplicated way as was easily understood and practised for maximum physical, mental and spiritual dividends. Also, the average yoga student needed to be convinced in his own scientific language that the process of yoga, or of any human action for that matter, is invariably a holistic one; one in which all the three coordinates—physical, mental and spiritual—come into play simultaneously in varying permutations and combinations. It follows then that any input at one plane unmistakably leaves its trail on 'the other two screens'. Viewed in this light ,the words 'health' and 'healing' assume much greater significance than is commonly appreciated. The verb 'to heal' actually means to 'make whole'. And to be whole or to be sound of health connotes much more than mere absence of pain, illness and symptoms. In its widest sense, it implies nothing less than correcting the course of destiny through the mechanism of an expanded and proactive consciousness. *Healing then, is not confined to the locus of your mind-body; healing actually means undoing the tormenting past and taming the uncertain future.*

All this eventually led me to take the final leap. Two other considerations that helped me make up my mind were (a) my standing as a city-based civil servant gave me a certain advantage over say, an *ashram*-oriented *sadhu*, in reaching out to the intelligentsia, and (b) in my own humble perception, I stood somewhere down the middle in the 'spiritual band' which had a *Siddha* at the one extreme and the yoga-initiate at the other. Given the nature of the project, one thing that

I have been determined to preserve at all costs, is authenticity. In detailing any account of the 'supernormal' phenomena, the temptation to exaggerate or dramatize is something that is hard to resist. In an age that thrives on marketing gimmicks, make- believe and sensationalism, my anxiety to cut out all frills and juicy story-telling might be slightly old-fashioned and, in the end, not particularly good commerce. At the end of the exercise however, I wanted to have the satisfaction of having steadfastly been honest and truthful in whatever I was describing. Accordingly, I make no claims to being anything like a yogi or even an exceptional seeker. Indeed, the main inspiration behind this book is my delight at having, as if by chance, discovered some of the greatest secrets of yoga that had, through God's inscrutable Will, chosen a down-to-earth person like me for their theatre. Consciously and carefully at every stage, I have followed a two-pronged strategy when describing the 'supernormal'—firstly, to put into the crucible my own experiences of the yogic phenomena before confidently revealing them to the reader and secondly, to rigidly stick to a first hand account of the 'still higher spiritual experiences' that were exclusively the preserve of *Siddhas* (on the rare occasion when I have found myself perched in the no man's land with neither my own experience nor a Siddha's teachings to guide me on the interpretation of any particular aspect of yoga, I have avoided becoming judgemental with a 'know all attitude', preferring instead to place all relevant facts before the discerning reader and encouraging him to 'be his own light'). On these two engines of knowledge, I have reposed trust as I voyage into the land of the unknown—some would say, the unknowable. While doing so, I have drawn inspiration from the *Vedic* and *Upanishadic* wisdom that, much as I would have liked to believe otherwise, is in fact not a product of fallible reason but is divinely 'revealed'. A die-hard skeptic in the initial years and then an agnostic in the interlude, I had additionally set but one condition for myself before I ventured into any such writing—that in course of my *Sadhana* or meditation, I must access and accumulate enough of genuine, first hand experience of the *Yoga 'miracles'* as find mention in scriptures and allied texts, to give my writings a ring of conviction. At this point of time when miracles have begun to truly flower in my life by the Grace of my Siddha Guru, I have run out of all excuses to dodge this 'responsibility'.

A miracle is defined as, "*an event or action that apparently contradicts known laws and is hence thought to be due to supernormal causes, specially to an act of God*". I leave it to the judgment of my esteemed readers as to which part of my experiences can be construed as resulting from scientifically explainable phenomena, and which part enters the realms of the 'miraculous'. By their very nature, spiritual experiences, specially the overtly 'supernormal' ones, are a very sacred and private affair between the seeker and the Almighty to be normally not divulged. On the other hand, it is sometimes the divine Will that a higher truth stumbled upon by an unsuspecting customer must, through him be relayed to the millions who believe and doubt in turns, and need reinforcement in this predicament. The purpose of giving a brief and functional description of my own experiences at the outset is neither to impress the reader with my yogic 'exploits', nor to convey the impression of my being any different from the vast multitude of theists, non-believers or the agnostics. Time and again in the book, I would be returning to the theme of how an ordinary seeker like me, blessed by a Siddha Guru and fortified by a strong will, could climb the first few steps of the dizzy heights of Yoga to get to know some of the fascinating realities 'on the other side of the fence'. In any case, psychic experiences or paranormal abilities do not rank too highly among the spiritual achievements, going by yoga theory, and are best ignored. These experiences however, serve a crucial purpose in keeping the seeker interested in the magnificently healing journey of yoga, with conspicuous milestones arriving at every meanwhile.

These are then some of the things that I have experienced chronologically in the last few years of my yoga practice:

1. Within first two months of sustained meditation, my chronic stomach disorders including indigestion, nausea and a duodenal ulcer disappeared completely.
2. With markedly reduced stress levels, came a new found appetite and new flesh that took my body-weight from a miserable 50 kgs (height—172 cm) to a much healthier 65 kgs.
3. With less irritability and aggression, there was this new found exuberance and interest in things around that led to a marked improvement in family ties and social interaction.
4. My face, specially the eyes, regained much of the old lustre that I had lost way back in my early 20's owing to stress and waywardness.
5. With the body having largely regained health, the inner energy or *Shakti* made its first visible exertions. I started feeling a kind of pleasant sensation at the space between the eyebrows during meditation.
6. During deep meditation, my body felt light like a cotton-ball. I could actually feel a buoyant energy building up in my lower back and surging up in waves to fill the back of my head.
7. My capacity and inclination to meditate increased markedly, so much so that any meditation session lasting less than one hour left me thirsting for more.
8. Each time after meditating, I tended to talk less (contrary to my normal talkative self!) and be much more relaxed, centred and vibrant for the rest of the day, savouring the tingling sensations that seemed to linger.
9. With the inner energy working ever more powerfully, the various *hatha-yogic asanas* that I had so far found difficult to perform, now came in a natural flow with a vigour, rhythm and pattern of their own.

10. A flurry of "supernormal" experiences that ensued, was enough to convince me that the *Kundalini-shakti*, the *chakras*, the *nadis* and the *koshas*—entities of the astral plane that are so meticulously described in scriptures and yoga classics—are all for real, and not metaphors as suggested by some 'secular' yoga theorists, specially in the West.

    The *Markandeya-Purana* mentions the following as the first signs of spiritual progress: enthusiasm, health, gentleness, pleasant odour, scant excretion, radiance and softness of voice. The *Yoga-Tattva-Upanishad* lists four external signs of *nadi-shuddhi* or purification of the pranic channels: bodily lightness (*laghava*), radiance (*dipti*), 'abdominal fire' (*jathara-agni*) and bodily shapeliness. The truth behind these scriptural observations had begun to dawn upon me in a very rapid, palpable and exhilarating turn of events. Compared to this, such startling 20th century findings as researcher Robert Wallace's (1978) that '*each year of regular meditation takes off roughly one year from your biological age*', seemed to be both elementary and unidimensional !

If the above description sounds impressive beyond credence, let me assure you once again that in the yoga theory, these are but the elementary signs of *Kundalini* awakening. The actual spiritual experiences of the higher kind are outwardly much less 'moving' and come only, if they come at all in one life, with many more years of meditation. The *Shiva–Samhita* tells us that there are all together four categories of yoga-practitioners : (a) the "mild practitioner" is dull-witted, wavering and a miracle-monger, (b) the "middle level" practitioner is poised, soft-spoken and of moderate habits, (c) the "ardent practitioner" is disciplined, energetic, compassionate and filled with faith, d) the "most ardent practitioner" is zealous, fearless, virtuous; knowing scriptures. While at the one extreme, the mild practitioner may take 12 years or more of sustained practice to succeed in yoga, the most ardent practitioner at the other end of the spectrum, may take less than 3 years to become a yoga adept. Clearly then, no tailor-made yoga standards can apply mechanically to all situations and all people. It is however axiomatic that the most consummate spiritual experiences, of which I can speak only on the strength of my understanding of scriptures, involve opening of the higher and still higher *chakras* or astral 'lotus centres'. They are directed largely at Self-Realization and are less concerned with relatively more 'earth-bound' considerations such as physical well-being and personality development. Here is then a more detailed account of what happened all this while in my rendezvous with Yoga.

"The mind is restless no doubt, and difficult to curb,
Arjuna; but it can be brought under control
by repeated practice
(of meditation) and by the exercise of dispassion,
O son of Kunti"

(*Gita*, 6:35)

I. The Transition

"I am still an atheist, thank God."

—Alfred Bunn

The Beginning

Over the last four years of serious meditation, I and those around me have seen the nearly miraculous effects that yoga, albeit of the esoteric kind, has had over my mind and body. In the early twenties and into my first job as a Grade A officer in NABARD, I carried a sickly frame of 45 kgs. And a mind so highly strung that it tended to go off in a tangent at the slightest emotional provocation or perceived injustice either to myself or to those around. Things became worse when, into my second job, I had the first real brush with people who mattered. The sheer hypocrisy, the near-perfect double standards, the subtle deceit and the crude arrogance—all this was proving to be just too much for a 'straight guy' like me; so much so that it started eating into my vitals. Given to recurrent bouts of emotional trauma and impotent rage in a very hostile environment, I developed a peptic ulcer in the mid 20s, something that won't let me have a single cup of tea or one morsel of solid food without causing vomiting. Although things did improve somewhat in the next 7-8 years, my health and psyche were badly dented and very much vulnerable to sudden pressures of circumstances. It was at this precarious stage of my life, when 'all seemed to be over', that I rather fortuitously, bumped into astrology, mysticism and yoga. A close friend of mine (whom I would call 'X') who happens to be a good astrologer and quite scholarly even otherwise, analysed my birth horoscope and made this startling prediction that I (the philistine !) was passing through a turning point in my life—Venus/Rahu—which would take me deeper and deeper into meditation and spiritualism. For my mundane problems that were seemingly converging on me from all corners, he suggested that I recite the *Aditya Hrdaya Stotra* (Hymn to Sun God) every morning, meditate as often as possible and take to vegetarianism to the extent I could.

One thing led to another till I was seriously into yoga and meditation. Through a rare coincidence, I also happened to lay my hands upon some breathtaking, yet down-to-earth literature on yoga and spiritualism. Among the most notable books that I read during those days of introspection and soul-searching were *'Autobiography of a Yogi'*, by Paramahansa Yogananda—the great *Siddha* of modern times in the footsteps of Vivekananda, *'Ramakrishna and his Disciples'* by the noted English novelist, Christopher Isherwood and *'Yogis, Destiny and the Wheel of Time'* by K. N. Rao—the internationally known bureaucrat–turned astrologer–turned spiritualist. As a student of English literature and philosophy during my academic days, I had had exposure to some quality literature ranging from the lilting poetry of Milton and Shelley to the lucid prose of Shaw and Lawrence. Without taking away from the obvious greatness of these legends, I can now vouchsafe that nothing touched my inner core the way these other worldly books did. Reading these books felt like touching live electric wires—a kind of earthquake taking place deep inside me that threatened to change everything, from my inner realms to the whole world order. Around that very period. I, till then a hard-core nonvegetarian who also relished an occasional peg in the company of close friends, seriously took to vegetarianism and teetotalism. Although neither I nor those whom I consulted on these matters had a puritanical outlook, I had gathered enough insight on the subject by this time to conclude that what one ate and drank had definite bearings on what one felt and 'became' in the long run.

Within two months of regular meditation, together with silent recital of the sacred Sanskrit hymn to Sun God, my peptic ulcer was completely healed, my chronic indigestion gone, my emotional state more resilient and most conspicuously, my body weight increased by a full four kgs, without any incremental food–intake or muscle-building exercises! (It was much later that I read authentic medical texts describing the pronounced anti-ageing and anabolic effects of sustained meditation on one's physique.) Inexplicably, but unmistakably I felt less at odds with the world around and in the next few months my dull and listless eyes began to glisten as they had never before. Another six months of regular meditation saw me experiencing even better physical and mental health and laid the foundations for a virtuous cycle of more meditation→leading to more quiescence→leading to more meditation. Exactly as has been described in the great books on the ancient Wisdom, I was inexplicably but surely experiencing a kind of inner balance and calm that had all my life been so alien to me. Until that time I had been used to spending sleepless nights brooding over lost career opportunities and family troubles. And although things outside remained much the same, I was somehow experiencing a high that was difficult to comprehend. I did not understand it then, but in retrospect I would sum it up simply this way—*I was being healed.*

Shortly after, as if through a divine design, I had the rare good fortune of coming in the contact of Yogi Hans Baba of Devraha lineage. My burgeoning interest in the paranormal had by this time taken me deep into probing the ethereal nature of the human form, the mystical working of mantra and the *Kundalini*-energy on the astral planes. In a leap of faith, I took *diksha* (mantra initiation) from Hans Baba, whom I was to only later recognize as a great *Siddha*. Under the seemingly divine inspiration of the great Guru, my meditation gained in depth and intensity. Often, meditating in the lotus posture or lying down in *shavasana*, I would get tingling sensations in the back and the scalp that are said to be the first signs of the activated *Kundalini* or the *pranic* energy powerhouse (in the years that followed, specially after my transfer from Patna to Delhi, I was fortunate enough to come in much greater physical contact with Hans Baba, and this added a whole new chapter to my forays in Yoga and the "supernormal"). The outer manifestation of it was that I was becoming more and more poised and centred even though the external environment continued to be adverse, often testing my limits. All this is not to suggest that I had overnight acquired the looks or the bearings of a yogi; I continue to be a very ordinary mortal and do not see myself, at this stage, becoming an adept in this life. The whole purpose however is to underline this eternal wisdom that you and I are, in essence no different from the Yogi, and the Yogi in turn is no different from God. And the yogic path that one so often and so casually takes just for fitness or 'as a nice way to relax' is in fact, quite unknown to him, his passport to much higher realms where health, peace and realization are not goals in themselves but the very nature of things.

At this stage I wish to recount two seemingly trivial incidents of my life. One pertains to the time when I was a teenager and the other, just before I took my second job in the Civil Services. In the first incident, I saw hundreds of fowls being slaughtered for meat at a picnic spot for 1st January celebrations, of which I was a participant. Although myself an avid meat-eater at that time, I felt so repulsed by the sight of bloodied flesh and feathers dispersed all around that I gave up meat-eating from that moment. Little did I realize that I had bitten more than I could chew. The next one year or so was of intense conflict and turmoil. The mere smell or sight of non-vegetarian food cooking, tickled my nostrils and fired my imagination; it then needed all my willpower to keep me from going back on my resolve. Things went on this tense and uneasy way till inevitably I reverted to my old and 'natural ' way of eating. The gentle persuasions of a friend one cold night during a hill-station outing afforded the fig–leaf for me to indulge in one bite, then another, and another....I took to eating meat with even greater relish and vengeance than before thereafter.

The other incident is somewhat hilarious but for its potentially serious career implications for me at the material time. As already described, I was extremely skinny and emaciated in my youth, going into my first job. Things had not changed much when I qualified for the coveted IAS and Allied Services in 1985 and braced up for the physical tests that were supposed to be more of a formality. I was allotted the Indian Railway Traffic Service which was supposed to be a very prestigious and challenging service, involving as it did the overseeing of train operations, revenue management and other mainstream activities. Since the IRTS, like the Indian Police Service, is supposed to be a very 'masculine' service calling for a lot of physical/outdoor activities, there is a prescribed minimum laid down for body-weight and chest-measurements for this service just as in the IPS. These minimums nevertheless, in the usual circumstances, are of token importance only, being liberal enough to let everyone pass them with the 'minimum' fuss. Or so it seemed till it was my turn to appear for the tests. To my and every one else's surprise, my 'exceptional' physique earned the rare distinction of failing these tests and promptly I got disqualified. All my dreams of joining an elite service seemed to be crashing around me for a reason that was as much comical as tragic.

After overcoming the early trauma, I sensed that there was one last hope. I could, under the provisions, still make a representation to an Appellate Medical Board within two months, and in the unlikely event of gaining ten kgs in weight and six cms in chest measurement, could give myself another shot at the physical test in order to be yet cleared for the particular service. The task seemed hopeless and my worst fears in this regard were confirmed by all the Patna based gymnasiums and medical experts. They were unanimous that it was not only impossible but also dangerous for me to try and gain 10 kgs in weight and 6 cms. in chest–width at such a short notice. Crestfallen and deeply resentful of my own puny frame that was so utterly lacking in muscles and fat, I somehow gathered myself and made a resolve—as was my wont—not to give up without a fight. Luckily, even with this figure, I had been a keen sportsman right from the childhood and therefore, physical exercise came naturally to me once I set my mind to it. For the next two months, it was all push-ups, jogging and the quickfix bulworker exercises alternated with ravenous consuming of dozens of *chapatis* and loads of *desi ghee*. During these two months, I worked at it like a man possessed and presto! I was a new man! My quantum leap in body weight and muscles was so big and dramatic that, aside from passing the physical tests, I gave my family and friends plenty to think and jest about. My eldest sister, Ratna, who lived in Sindri at that time, happened to arrive at our Patna residence one early morning and on being told that I was still sleeping on the terrace, climbed upstairs only to balk back. In her own words, "it was not the lean and thin me but some very robust and manly looking stranger sleeping out there with the face pressed against the pillow" My boundless joy at having passed the physical re-examination through such an unlikely turn of events had an added dimension in that I now revelled in my new-found physical and social stature. Friends who till the other day were used to making fun of my 'mini-frame', began to awe and marvel at my manly figure and occasionally touched the finely chiselled sinews that appeared to have popped up almost overnight from nowhere. Sadly this fairy tale was short-lived. Once the immediate objective of passing the Civil Services medical test was met, I sub-consciously lost the drive and gradually relapsed into my old routine of physical lethargy and irregular meals. This coupled with recurrent attacks of dysentery ensured that I was almost back to my 'original self'.

It did not occur to me then; but at this juncture, I feel there is a lot to learn from these two 'stray' incidents of my life. In both the instances, my good intents were backed by an unusually strong will to succeed, and consequently brought about remarkable success in the short run. However, this almost overnight success was a painful, contrived and lop-sided exercise in self-denial that did not take care of the fundamentals, with the result that success was superficial and short-lived. The purely physical approach that I was driven to adopt in either instance under the compulsion of circumstances was bound to fail, even boomerang, no matter how strongly pursued. For the forces that underlie and shape man's tastes, temperament and physique go much deeper than one's physical body. They are rooted in one's soul as it were, and are as such bound to return sooner or later with increased vehemence. "Pluck not the leaves, but treat the roots if you want to avoid the bitter harvest"—seems to be the moral of my two stories. How fascinatingly my approach in the two incidents of my youth contrasts with my own inner rearranging in the later phase when, simply meditating and without even knowing what exactly to expect or aspire for, I saw my urge to eat meat, take liquor as also my skinniness gradually diminish, and finally wear off without any trying or internal conflict!

The Goa Miracle

All this appeared to be nothing short of a miracle, more to my family members and intimate friends than to myself, because unlike me, they had no idea of what was going on inside me. Yet my psycho-physical metamorphosis over the last few years fell tantalizingly short of my own yardstick to measure the 'supernormal'. The skeptic within me now yearned for a more conclusive proof of the divine. I continued my meditation sessions in the coming years despite occasional hiccups and lows. Then recently, during one of my outstation visits, I had another glimpse of what lies on the 'other side of the fence'. For last many years, I have intermittently had this problem of spondylites–like attacks—pulled back-muscles and frozen shoulders that would hurt excruciatingly at the slightest movement of the upper torso and would virtually incapacitate me for several days for that reason. In the past whenever this occurred, I had to seek either the doctor's help or the services of the traditional 'bone setters', with largely unsatisfactory and temporary results. During this visit—at one of the places in Goa—I was looking forward to lots of sight-seeing amidst my tight schedule, and here I was, bed-ridden and sulking, with a full-blown onset of the old problem. I was in a fix and getting nervous in the alien land. What could I do now?

Of late I had been reading some books on Reiki; its efficacy and versatility as delineated in the writings was still fresh in my memory. I wished I knew Reiki myself and wondered if there could be some Reiki practitioner around who could possibly help me out of this awkwardness (ironically, I was to become a full-fledged Reiki Master soon after, and in an inspired burst, became instrumental in dramatic healing of many friends and relatives, at least one of which was a near terminal case with the doctors having given up all hope! But that is another story altogether). Then I uncertainly reasoned, that the underlying principle of both Reiki and Yoga was one and the same—drawing from the infinite pool of the all-pervasive Cosmic Energy that was universally healing and illuminating. If Reiki could work for me, I figured out, then yoga might as well do the trick. Till then I had benefited from the efficacy of yoga in removing physiological disorders of a more general nature in a gently unfolding way. But here I was up against a very specific and acute physical disability that called for immediate relief. What gave me heart was that I had now been meditating for roughly three years. And I had the added advantage of being spiritually initiated, thus being able to meditate with the aid of what is called a "*Chaitanya mantra* " *i. e.,* mantra enlivened and charged with the yogic powers of a *Siddha* who has so to say, taken your ordinary frame under his wings through the rather mysterious process of *diksha.* Promptly I sat meditating in the lotus posture—*Padmasana*—somehow trying to ignore the pain and the stiffness. Till then, in the usual course I meditated with the silent repetition of the Mantra for about three-quarters of an hour in one go. In this instance however, I kept meditating and meditating in a part-curious part-desperate bid to make something happen. I was encouraged by the same inner tingling sensation that appears to rise in waves in the lower back and finds its way up my scalp and forehead during my regular meditation-sessions, but which now felt as if it was hitting the exact spasm-locations and the nerve-blockages with a cascade of energy-shafts. I got up after a good two hours or thereabouts. The result was amazing—bordering on the miraculous. Without my touching the sore back, shoulder or neck muscles, my problem had vanished altogether in a matter of two hours. Something that used to pin me down for weeks in spite of the best medical care was cured in two hours flat by sheer mind power! After this discovery of sorts, I have still had back-spasms and frozen shoulders on a couple of occasions (something that I suspect has largely to do with my bad postures during sleep and long hours of TV watching) but each time I have been able to fight it off the same way: meditating. For me this was another instance of mind spectacularly triumphing over matter.

The Dawn

All this was slowly convincing me at the intellectual level that there was much more to our existence than science and 'rationality' would admit. Meanwhile, Newtonian notions of mass and energy along with the age-old Cartesian dualism of mind and matter had already ceased to be sacrosanct. Quantum physicists were emulating scriptures in boldly asserting the existence of a Unified Energy Field—a Supreme Consciousness—underlying all events and existence, and of the ever pulsating mind-matter flux. But these adventures and speculations apart, I still longed for a more direct confrontation with the 'supernormal' so as to give a firmer ground to my nascent forays into metaphysics that were yet rooted in pragmatism.

Finally, I was able to lay my hands on a series of 'experiences'—more concrete, convincing and unquestionably 'supernormal'—through the Grace of Hans Baba. A lot has been written about this great yogi of the classical Patanjali tradition including a biography of him by K. N. Rao that has one article contributed by novelist Amrita Pritam describing her miraculous cure. I wish to write about the Guru and my series of mystical experiences under Baba's influence at a later stage. Meanwhile, this fascinating encounter with the transcendental state at last gave me the necessary courage and conviction to go about writing this present book.

In my whole exercise, I would consider my mission fulfilled if I am able to satisfactorily and correctly explain the basics of the theory and practice underlying the much misunderstood mechanics of yoga, meditation and mantra that are essentially the three sides of the same spiritual monolith. But at the outset I would like my reader to correctly understand the true meaning of some much abused expressions in this field. Unlike the popular belief, the Hindu scriptures –essentially the Vedas, the Upanishads and Yoga classics—pass muster as scientific texts in the sense that each term is exactly and uniquely defined, thus being incapable of different interpretations. Just as the seemingly like expressions of 'speed' and 'velocity' have unique and distinct meanings in Newtonian physics, similarly words such as *Yoga, Dhyana, Karma, Chitta* and so on, as occurring in the ancient texts, carry exact and unique meanings, thus being incapable of loose interpretations even in this era of masala-mix. To talk of ' *bhavatita dhyana*' or Transcendental Meditation is for example, to betray one's ignorance of the fact that *Dhyana* (Meditation) cannot be anything but *Bhavatita* (Transcendental). Similarly to dabble in some forced breathing exercises in the name of '*Pranayama*' is asking for trouble since *Pranayama*, bereft of its focus and perspective, is a double-edged weapon that can injure more than it can deliver.

We would see what Yoga actually means in the *Vedic* wisdom, in a short while. But in the next chapter I would like to get my reader to lower his guards of the so-called scientific temper, by juxtaposing the ancient theory of Yoga with some of the most sensational and insightful findings in the fields of quantum physics, new medicine and parapsychology. The growing body of scientific evidence that uncannily alludes to the essentially spiritual and holistic nature of man and the universe is part of the reason why the West has now taken the lead in rediscovering the seemingly archaic theories contained in the ancient Hindu scriptures. As the frontiers of particle physics and metaphysics are tending to merge imperceptibly, there is now a strong case for the intellectually most gifted to take the resurgent yoga movement to its logical culmination of mind-body-spirit unity, for the greatest individual and common good.

To Recap

1. Mind has primacy over matter and therein lie the great secrets of yoga.
2. Modern science and ancient scriptures are one in asserting the existence of a Unified Energy Field—a Supreme Intelligence—underlying all phenomena.
3. Best breathing is natural breathing; pranayama practice bereft of its perspective, injures more than it heals.

4. The yoga-path, so often casually taken by practitioners for fitness and relaxation is, unknown to them, their passport to higher realms of Realization .
5. The apparently biological forces underlying man's tastes, temperament and physique are rooted in the soul, and can be neutralized only by 'soul force'.

II. The Science of Yoga

"If you want to see real psycho–kinesis, then consider the facts of mind-over–matter performed in the brain. It is quite astonishing that with every thought, the mind manages to move the atoms of hydrogen, carbon, oxygen, and the other particles in the brain's cells."

—SIR JOHN ECCLES (*Nobel Prize Winning Neurologist*)

Yoga and the Times

The first thoughts that come to mind at the mention of the word "Yoga" are not easy to define. Is it meditation and mind control? Is it stretching, contraction and curling of the body in different shapes? Is it breath control and a fixed gaze? Is it chanting and observing silence? Yoga is in fact all this, and a lot more. An appreciation of the wide scope and complexity of yoga is possible simply by going through the names of different versions of yoga—*Hatha-yoga*, *Raja-yoga*, *Bhakti-yoga*, *Kundalini-yoga*, *Siddha-yoga*, *Laya-yoga*, and so on. What the Westerner however is likely to readily identify yoga with, is a set of static and dynamic physical postures/exercises—more specifically, '*Hatha-yoga*'.

The concept of yoga as a natural extension of the Indian philosophical tradition was first introduced to Westerners by the redoubtable Vivekananda. Its practicable and utilitarian dimension was then carried to the West by Paramahansa Yogananda in early twentieth century in the form of *Kriya-yoga* with a relatively greater emphasis on breathing and psycho-technical methods. From that point onwards, there has been an ever growing tendency in the West to make yoga almost synonymous with *Hatha-yoga.* Twisting and curling, stretching and bending—the classic body postures of yoga are now an integral part of the typical modern yoga centre, both in the West and in cosmopolitan India. They seem to fit more easily into our physically inclined society, and the larger part of yoga's appeal in these times stems from its now proven ability to chisel and cure the body in today's cult of physical fitness.

Yet, *hatha-yoga* is a relatively late addition in the yoga tradition, dating from about the 10th Century AD. Given its mass appeal and wide acceptability, it is interesting to note that *hatha-yoga* is a relatively more difficult form of yoga-practice calculated to tap assiduously a whole gamut of dormant energies lying in wait inside the body. Cleansing (*Kriyas*), purifying (*Shodhana*), breath manipulation (*Pranayama*) and an astounding range of physical postures (*Asana*)—all designed to unleash the primal life-force(*Prana*)—together comprise *hatha-yoga. Hatha-yoga* was, therefore, always intended for those who already possessed reasonable bodily strength. Besides, it called for the help of an adept teacher, at least to begin with. Any attempt to do too much too soon or test one's limits, however tempting, must be scrupulously avoided. 'Yoga injuries' occur more in *hatha-yoga* practice, than in any other mode of yoga–pursuit thanks to its physicality and athleticism. There is no denying however, that the *hatha-yoga* practice when done properly in moderation and under expert guidance, removes stress and tones up the physique. The regular *hatha-yoga* practitioner however, would do well to avoid fixation with the body, and should rather be on the look out for the attending benefits on the mental and spiritual levels. As a matter of fact, scriptures testify that the whole science of hatha-yoga came about through the seers' close observation of those spiritual men who were experincing a powerful surge of the Kundalini under the Divine influence. The seers found out that a systamatic replication of those yogic postures and seals could in turn, aid awakening of the *kundalini* with all attendant benfits. Increased self-confidence, inner poise and emotional highs are not infrequently reported.

For the yoga aspirants who are less physically endowed, the *hatha-yoga* path may not hold much promise. The yoga spectrum nevertheless, has numerous other options which can be synthesized for safe and optimum gains. *Jnana-yoga*—the path of intellectual development, *Karma-yoga*—the path of service, *Mantra-yoga*—the path that works on sound/thought vibrations, *Raja-yoga*—the essentially psychological discipline of stilling the turbulent thought processes, *Tantra*—the yoga that makes use of symbols and rituals; all these are yogic pathways that can be suitably adopted with an eye on the mental and the spiritual. Physical well-being, in any case, is a natural offshoot of mental and spiritual health and is therefore likely to come naturally to the yoga practitioner even without conscious pursuit of *hatha-yoga*.

Yoga and 'Health'

In Latin, if we recall, *to heal* means *to make whole*. Accordingly, health means not mere absence of physical disease, but a certain 'wholeness' of existence extending symmetrically in all three dimensions—physical, mental and spiritual. Insofar as yoga is said to promote health, it has to, by definition, address much larger concerns than the human physique. One would also recall that the tendency to think of yoga merely in terms of physical fitness and mind–relaxation was likened to grossly under-utilizing a PC as a typewriter. In essence, yoga is a spiritual discipline emanating from man's deepest desires to break loose of the nitty-gritty of mundane existence. It was then, meant to facilitate the human effort to identify with something of transcendental nature and significance—something that could underpin our own finite and fragile existence. For the perfectionist, yoga therefore, is a means to employ the distilled wisdom of the Indian philosophical heritage in such manner as to make him rise above all polarities of life and death, mind and body, joy and sorrow, togetherness and separation.

What then becomes of the yoga–craving of the average Westerner who fancied yoga as something that could make him feel better, sleep better, and in the bargain, got him rid of a few addictions? How does the grandiose concept of a Supreme and Unified Consciousness (the word 'yoga' literally means 're-union') go hand in hand with a rather modest desire to say no to the bottle or to tackle a stiff back? Much of the apparent dichotomy however, goes away if we reflect that the yearning for cosmic re-union that engages man outwardly, is but a mirror–reflection of the struggle within to achieve a certain inner unity at the micro level. Bereft of this inner union, we mostly remain at odds with ourselves—torn asunder and shoved about by the conflicting pulls and pressures of life that have less to do with reason than with our basic instincts. The mind in the waking state is estimated to experience over 50,000 random thoughts each day, a majority of them directed at the conflicting, the absurd or the impossible. The physical body, attempting to respond to this chaos, chokes and maladapts to cause illness. Most of our energy is wasted thus, as the mind self-destructs. If on the other hand, the 'monkey mind' is somehow got rid of bulk of these 50,000 subterranean thoughts at their source—a bundle of our habits, complexes and defences—the energy of consciousness thus compacted, gains the necessary momentum to travel up the spine and, one by one, vivify the hidden psycho-energetic vortices to usher in healing, awareness and bliss.

Unlike clinical psychology, yoga with its holistic approach, goes beyond the psychological process and rearranges our primal life forces enabling us to achieve an inner unity within ourselves; encouraging us to be in closer contact with our inner core and drawing sustenance from its new found solidity and roundness. As soon as this inner cohesion discovers itself and begins to flower, all negativity and defensiveness starts gradually falling off. Having tapped your own inner reservoirs, you suddenly find that the urge to smoke, drink or eat unhealthily has tapered off on its own. Consequently, you get rid of your bad habits without the usual inner conflict. In other words, *you do not give up the bad habits; it is the bad habits that 'give you up'*. Not surprisingly, yoga which till the seventies, was thought of as largely the preserve of renunciates who would have nothing of this world, increasingly thereafter penetrated the West. The Westerners began understanding this great secret of the Eastern tradition, that the yoga–adept 'disinvested' in order that he got back more of everything!

In keeping with the holistic nature of all influences, accessing an inner sense of unity is often accompanied by a marked rejuvenation of the stressed and diseased body. It is also quite often accompanied by a pronounced improvement in family ties and greater poise in social relations. Simultaneously, yoga's net effect of turning you inward means that the highs and lows of external living seem to no longer hold the same old bite.

Yoga and Medicine

The Medical Revolution

Towards the middle of the nineteenth century, virtually every field of knowledge was undergoing cataclysmic changes, including the science of medicine. Louis Pasteur, a French Scientist, gave currency to the modern germ theory. Very quickly, it came to be acknowledged that we live in a world teeming with animate micro-organisms that among other things, produced infective diseases. Subsequently Dr. Robert Koch, a German doctor, identified the specific bacteria responsible for cholera and tuberculosis. As the 20th century dawned, Alexander Fleming discovered penicillin. This miracle–medicine enabled millions to escape death and suffering caused by a host of bacterial diseases. 'Extraneous' considerations such as diet, patient's life-style and attitude, were weeded out; a penicillin shot did the trick regardless. Increasingly, treatment became disease-centred rather than patient-oriented. The patient did not figure at all in the healing process, and was rather, a receptacle of antimicrobial drugs and procedures. Antibiotics, vaccines allied with vastly improved public sanitation and living standards led to a substantially hiked average life expectancy. Modern medicine, together with its practitioner, accordingly grew manifold in stature and acceptability, till it became an empire. The Allopathic system, now holding centre-stage and having elbowed out all competition, was to become the last word in medical treatment. 'Allopathy', derived from the Greek, *allopatheia* that means "subject to external influences," banked on procedures that elicit effects opposite that of the disease. Antibiotics, anti-inflammatories, antifungals and like other drugs became the rage. Removing symptoms without concern for the underlying causes was all that engaged the physician. Very soon, doctors graduating from "scientific" medical schools were the only ones who could legally practise medicine. In a post–industrial revolution world-civilization whose imagination was increasingly getting fired by scientific breakthroughs, allopathy was easily able to subjugate traditional medicinal systems with its scientific appeal. Each illness was now paired with a particular cause; the notion of mind influencing the body that had dominated ancient and medieval medicine faded into oblivion. The 'placebo effect', then made way for far more invasive techniques.

Placebo; the Second Revolution

As research continued, the scientific community however, came to this uneasy realization that a patient's trust in his doctor is still crucial. Research further showed that the doctor's own orientation towards the patient and towards his own methods, had decisive bearing on the results of his treatment. Beyond doubt, it now transpired that allopaths, like the shamans, gained enormously from the body's latent ability to subdue most physical diseases that asserted itself in the right conditions. Studies also showed that several subtle, seemingly trivial variables, such as the doctor's attention/ reputation, the colour of pills, the mode of administering the drug (injections or capsules), the size and count of tablets, and so on, decisively influenced the outcome of all allopathic treatment.

A double-blind study was undertaken in mid 20th century involving patients of *angina pectoris.* Surgeons performed pseudo operations in which the patients "knew" that their arteries were being tied off to increase blood supply to the heart muscles. In reality however, the arteries were only surgically opened and then simply closed again! Startlingly enough, results showed that the "sham" surgery had turned out to be as effective as real surgery, and in some trials, gave even better results. In decades that followed, pseudo-surgery was increasingly employed to yield significant success in such varied conditions as Perkinson's disease and arthritis. These 'operations' were roundly criticized by the medical orthodoxy as unethical on account of the risks involved—sedation, infection and post-operative complications. At the other extreme, with recent technological advancements making surgery less and less invasive, a significant number of medical researchers came to view 'sham surgery' as a standard surgical technique usable in a variety of conditions where conventional surgery was precluded for one or the other reason.

In another group of studies, dummy drugs administered to a group of cancer patients in the garb of strong chemotherapy, induced typical side-effects of chemotherapy, complete with extreme nausea and hair loss! In 1980s, Evelyn Silvers, a Los Angeles based therapist carried out a milestone study involving 20 hard-core drug addicts. All these patients were hopelessly dependent on alcohol, valium, heroin or cocaine. The addiction, in all these cases, was serious enough to have ravaged their physique, family-life and social adjustment. Silvers psyched the patients into believing that the brain's inner pharmacy had enough "natural drugs" in store to satisfy them and overcome any disorder, including excruciating pain. Next, the subjects were asked to close their eyes and visualize that each of them was creating inside the head, a supply of neurochemicals that were the "originals" mimicked by the artifical drugs; storing and building it up to a critical threshold.

As the subjects mentally pictured with closed eyes, a sizeable build-up of the equivalent of their favoured drugs, and finally 'injected' it into their blood stream when she signalled, a miracle happened. Each of the drug addicts experienced a massive drug–high that replicated his own, accustomed upswing with the abuse of valium, cocaine or one of these substances. From this discovery, de-addiction was only a small step away for these participants, since they were now shown to be masters, rather than slaves of the drugs. Earlier, Silvers had used the same guided visualization technique to get a group of patients to internally produce *endorphine*, the most powerful of pain killers, so as to ease symptoms of arthritis, migraine and lower back-pain.

Truly, no state of mind exists without a corresponding biochemical plank. A gamut of studies has now conclusively demonstrated the powerful hold of the placebo on man's psyche and physique. The dictionary definition of 'placebo' as *"a harmless, unmedicated preparation given as a medicine to a patient merely to humour him..."* is now increasingly seen to be unsatisfactory. The word itself is derived from the Latin *placere*, meaning "to please". The placebo, which essentially refers to the powerfully intervening psychological aspects of the patient's treatment, was greatly valued in traditional medicine, then upstaged and nearly uprooted by allopathy; only to come back with a vengeance in the second half of the 20th century. Thomas Dolbanco, M.D.—an associate professor of medicine at Harvard Medical School—testifies:

> "*....The placebo is one of the most powerful medicines we have. It's very hard to tell sometimes whether what we're doing is more than the placebo effect....*"

Andrew Weil—the best-selling author of '*Spontaneous Healing*' who happens to be a graduate from Harvard Medical School and now Director of the Programme in Integrative Medicine at the University of Arizona, favours a reform of medical education with some suggestions as below:

(a) Exposure to the philosophy of science based on quantum physics bypassing the antiquated concepts of Newtonian mechanics and Cartesian dualism.
(b) Recognition of nature's own healing mechanisms and mind/body interactions including placebos and psychoneuroimmunology.
(c) Guidance in spirituality and psychology together with conceptual models explaining physical events as arising from non-physical actions.
(d) Basic understanding of alternative medicine.
(e) Instruction in meditation, guided imagery and visualisation techniques.

Exactly how the placebo and spiritual techniques work is not yet understood by medical science. In *Spontaneous Remission*, researchers O'Regan and Hirshberg recognize an innate healing mechanism operating within each person that appears to contain at least three components : (i) a Self-Diagnostic System, (ii) a Self-Repair System, and iii) a Regenerative System. These researchers also found that this kind of healing could be triggered by signals, suggestions and guidance from the physical, mental and/or spiritual realms of every individual.

Yoga and Physics

For last several centuries, the mystics' world view was forced to take the back seat, castigated by scientific realism that valued a fundamental distinction between the ultimate constituents of the universe. This classical view has now however, been overturned. New Age science comes periliously close to the mystical concept of reality as made up of interconnections and fusion, rather than as comprised of 'basic building blocks'. The Einsteinean thesis—that everything existing could ultimately be traced to one force field—is strikingly yogic in its approach. The only major departure is that what remains an empty concept to modern science is a fact of everyday experience to the illumined yogi.

Fritjof Capra, author of the *Tao of Physics,* had this to say in his keynote address at the Los Angeles Symposium on Physics and Metaphysics, in 1977.

> *"My field is physics, a science which, in the 20th century, has led to a radical revision of many of our basic concepts of reality. For example, the concept of matter is very different in sub-atomic physics from the traditional idea of a material substance that was held in classical physics. The same is true of other concepts of reality such as space, time, objects or cause and effect. Out of these changes in our concepts of reality, a new world-view is emerging. This view turns out to be closely related to the views of mystics of all ages and traditions, particularly the religious philosophies of the Far East—Hinduism, Buddhism, Taoism....*
>
> *....In contrast to the mechanistic view of classical Western science, the Eastern view could be called an organic, holistic, or ecological view. Things and phenomena are perceived as being different manifestations of the same reality. The division of the world into separate objects, though useful and practical on the everyday level, is seen as an illusion—Maya, as the*

Indians say. To Eastern mystics, objects have fluid and ever-changing character. Change and transformation, flow and movement, play an essential role in their world-view. The cosmos is seen as one inseparable reality, forever in motion. It is alive, organic, spiritual and material at the same time. A very similar view is now emerging from modern physics....

....Quantum Theory showed that the sub-atomic particles have no meaning as isolated entities, but can only be understood as interconnections between various agencies of observation and measurement. Particles are not things but interconnections between things; and these things are interconnections between other things, and so on.

Quantum Theory thus reveals a basic oneness of the universe. It shows that we cannot decompose the world into independently existing smallest units. As we penetrate into matter, Nature does not show us any isolated basic building blocks, but rather appears as a complicated web of relations between the various parts of a unified whole.

This network of relations, furthermore, is intrinsically dynamic. According to Quantum Theory, matter is never quiescent, but always in a state of motion. Macroscopically, the materials around us may seem dead and inert. But if you magnify a piece of metal or stone, you realize that it is full of activity.

Modern physics pictures matter, not as passive and inert, but as continuously dancing and vibrating. This is very much like the Eastern mystics' description of the world. Both emphasize that the universe has to be grasped dynamically. Its structures are not static, rigid ones, but should be seen in terms of dynamic equilibrium.

Physicists speak of the continuous dance of sub-atomic matter which goes on all the time. They have actually used the words 'dance of creation and destruction' or 'energy dance'. This naturally comes to mind when you see some of the pictures of particles taken by physicists in their bubble chambers.

Of course, physicists are not the only ones talking about this cosmic dance. Perhaps the most beautiful example of this metaphor exists in Hinduism—the idea of the dancing Lord Siva. Siva is the personification of the cosmic dance. According to Indian tradition, all life is a rhythmic interplay of death and birth, of creation and destruction.... "

Not surprisingly then, Sir James Jeans has this to say in his *'The Mysterious Universe'—*

"The stream of knowledge is heading towards a non-mechanical reality; the universe begins to look more like a great thought than like a great machine."

As if the continuing assimilation of the new physics in classical yoga was not enough of a shock, the inaugural speech delivered by Sir J. C. Bose in the opening ceremony of the Bose's Institute way back in 1940s, contained this astounding observation—

"A universal reaction seemed to bring metal, plant and animal under a common law. They all exhibited essentially the same phenomena of fatigue and depression, with possibilities of recovery and of exaltation, as well as the permanent unresponsiveness associated with death."

It may perhaps be in order to end this chapter with this remarkable revelation from Krishna:

"Arjuna, whatsoever being, animate or inanimate, is born, know it as emanated from the union of Ksetra *(Matter) and the* Ksetrajna *(Spirit)."*

(*Gita,* 13:26)

To Recap

Yoga and the Times

1. The tendency in the West is to make yoga synonymous with physical *asanas*.
2. Physical *asanas* are only a fraction of yoga and a relatively late addition.
3. Yoga means 'reunion'—the lofty ideal of cosmic reunion is a mirror reflection of the struggle to achieve inner reunion.
4. The inner reunion, once achieved, sets off the healing process of yoga.
5. The verb 'To heal' literally means 'To make whole'; absence of inner chasms and not disease is the true sign of health.

Yoga and Medicine

6. Early twentieth century (allopathic) medicine was antagonistic in approach—antibiotic, anti-fungal, anti-inflammatory etc.
7. Patient was less a partner in the healing process and more a passive recipient
8. The doctor insisted that each illness could be traced to a specific cause, rejecting the notion that mind could influence body.
9. In 1950s, double-blind studies showed that sham surgery in heart diseases could be equally or more effective compared to 'the real thing'.
10. The placebo effect is now recognized as wonderful medication and the medical science now recognizes the mind–body flux.
11. There is now a move for reforming medical education so as to emphasize the inherent healing power of nature and body and include instruction on spirituality, psychology and alternative medicine.

Yoga and Physics

12. Modern science and Eastern mysticism lead to very similar views of the universe.
13. The concept of matter, time space, cause and effect in quantum physics is radically different from that in classical physics.
14. Quantum theory reveals a basic oneness of the universe and shows matter to be dancing and vibrating, rather than passive and inert.

III. Yoga in Perspective

"(Of God) The worst that can be said is that he's an under achiever."

— Woody Allen

The Twilight and After

The Sunrise-.... 5000 BC

We have now seen how the popular version of yoga that is practised today, specially in the West, is only the tip of the iceberg. In essence, it is ancient India's studied response to man's deep rooted spiritual thirst and existential questioning that could not be banished till this day despite all attempts to rid our largely materialistic culture of its mystical baggage. From the invisible, pre-historic roots in traditions akin to shamanism to the pluralistically unfolding contemplative cultures of Hinduism, Buddhism and Jainism, Yoga has gradually unfolded in India with such contemporariness as to now storm the sensitive and scientifically-inclined West. The manifest purpose of Yoga has been to study not the laws of matter, but the very fringes of consciousness. For, this Indian tradition was aware at all times that consciousness precedes energy, and energy underlies matter. For an esoteric system that is thousands of years old, this is a remarkably bold concept that as already seen, is now finding favour with modern physics and molecular biology. As the 20th century becomes history, an ever increasing number of discerning Westerners, not to speak of the Indian intelligentsia that in search of its values looks askance at the West, is gravitating to the East for spiritual succour and fulfillment. In the bargain, many have tentatively grasped the wonderful reconciliation of body and spirit that gradually occurs in encounters with Yoga. Far from engendering exclusivism or fundamentalism of any kind, Yoga has tended to take the practitioner towards a greater insight in his native faith and a responsible otherworldliness that transcends ideological prevarications.

The sheer versatility and historical expanse of Yoga makes it by far the forerunner among world's cherished traditions of psycho-spiritual upliftment. Historically, the Yoga tradition goes back to some 7000 years, although the clear outlines begin to emerge only around 1000 BC. Terracotta seals dating from the Indus Valley Civilisation depict figures recognizable as gods, sitting in various yoga postures. Among the yogic postures so depicted is the familiar lotus posture, with legs folded and crossed, hands resting on knees and the upper back erect.

The Vedas: 5000-2500 BC

The earliest proto-yogic themes and practices can be traced to the fountainhead of Hinduism, the Vedas. Unambiguously, there is evidence of metaphysical speculations in the *Rig Veda*, a collection of hymns that directly "descended" on ancient Indian "seers". Till recently, scholars were inclined to tentatively assign *Rig Veda*, the oldest of the four Vedas, to around 1500 BC. Recent research however has revealed this collection to be much older with evidence favouring its dating to 4000 BC or earlier. All subsequent *Vedic* literature has been dated back correspondingly. Swami Rama, the great yoga-adept of modern times, in his memoirs recalls that ancient *Tantric* manuscripts in original at least 4000 years old, were seen by him to be preserved in the *Gurukula* tradition, in the snowy Himalayan caves that were his abode for most of his adolescence. The famous oral tradition of preservation of scriptural knowledge that is the life-breath of

Hindu Thought must therefore, go back a few more millenniums by all accounts. This should be a sobering influence on the minds of those yoga-researchers and Indologists who tend to take the historical dates of yoga–evolution too literally. These historical dates serve their purpose more as probabilities and loosely defined ranges rather than watertight compartments.

Although seeds of Yoga germinated in the Indus Valley Civilisation, these peoples are said by modern historians to be in time, overrun by the Sanskrit speaking, presumably Indo-European *Vedic* tribes coming from the north. As mentioned, it is the *Vedic* era that actually gives us the first glimpses of yoga as we know. The concept of addressing and expanding one's awareness was an integral part of the *Vedic* concept of yoga and time and again *Vedic* hymns, starting with the *Rig Veda*, allude to esoteric practices that would today easily be called meditation. These *Vedic* hymns clearly speak of breath control, stilling the thought process by concentration and contemplation, and surrendering the ego in intense devotion as the means to abandoning the narrow self and experiencing the transcendental bliss. The hymns while enunciating the goal of Enlightenment also advanced speculative theories about the creation of the Universe. From the Yoga point of view, the most crucial hymnodies are the *Rig Veda* and the *Atharva Veda*. The *Atharva Veda* came a little after the *Rig Veda* and comprises magical incantations over and above hymns of metaphysical import.

The Upanishads: 1500–600 BC

The *Vedic* people envisaged formal rituals for effecting spiritual transformation. However, from about 1000 BC or before, a relatively more mystical trend surfaced in the form of the *Upanishads*. The *Upanishads* are among the most spiritually pregnant works of yoga which came to be known as the *Vedanta,* or the 'End of knowledge'. These comprise around 200 mystical writings that emphasize a less extroverted form of enlightenment. Contemplation and meditation continue to be the major planks of yoga practice, but these were now intended as means to forge links with an immanent, immutable Self at the core of man's being rather than with an external one. *Upanishadic* literature continued to take shape through many centuries. The earlier *Upanishads* did not address themselves to practical ways and means of ascent from ego–identity to Self–identity. Instead, Yoga is first spoken of in clear terms as a spiritual method in the *Kathopanishad*. Composed in the 6th century BC or before, this first truly yogic Upanishad propounds *adhyatma-yoga* or 'Yoga of the inmost self' that enabled the adept one to access the supreme Self at the nucleus of his own being.

Buddhisim and Jainism: 600 BC

It was around the 6th century BC that Buddhism took shape out of Buddha's teachings, founded in a spurning of all metaphysical speculation, specially the concept of an eternal indwelling Self. Buddha, a prince turned ascetic, made a major departure from the orthodox *Vedic* tradition. Interestingly ancient Hindu texts are believed to mention him (*Gautama* or *Siddhartha*) as the ninth incarnation of God. Some Sanskrit texts also refer to him as a *yogin*, i.e., a yoga adept. The Buddha emphasized a path of practical discipline which even after more than 2500 years, finds favour with millions of followers concentrated mainly in Asian countries, and which is now increasingly fascinating the West. Buddhism comprises eight correct psychophysical practices to be observed simultaneously. The ethical contents, the body postures and concentration techniques of Buddhism, including the much talked about *Vipassana*, are completely yogic in style.

Around that very time, another similar practice-oriented approach came about in the form of teachings of Vardhaman Mahavira, founder of Jainism. A slightly older contemporary of Buddha, Mahavira was the last in a chain of illumined ones. Together, Buddhism and Jainism had a profound impact on the further development of yoga, specially in its philosophical treatment that was carried forward by Patanjali, who would come much later.

The Epics: 300BC—200 AD

The two national epics that form the cornerstone of the Hindu way of living even in modern India, are the *Ramayana* and the *Mahabharata*. These two expansive stories, contain the quintessential yogic concepts and serve as important reference for yoga values and philosophy. The *Ramayana* came into existence around 3rd century BC after its author, Valmiki, notorious as a thief earlier, was so much reformed by meditation as to become a sage. In the *Ramayana*, Rama symbolizes the yogic qualities of ethical conduct, self-restraint and non-attachment, even while dispensing worldly obligations. Rama also happens to be regarded as the 7th incarnation of God, Vishnu in the Hindu tradition.

The *Mahabharata*, written down around the 2nd century AD, is the story of a War between two ancient ruling peoples, the Pandavas and the Kauravas that is reckoned to have been fought around 1000 BC. The *Mahabharata*, with its epic war, essentially symbolizes the struggle between good and evil. It is however, most significant for the fact that it contains the *Bhagavad Gita*. Although it is but an episode of the *Mahabharata*, the *Bhagavad Gita* is a complete yoga text in itself, and regarded by many as arguably the greatest spiritual work ever known to mankind. The most famous of all yoga scriptures, this 'Lord's Song', consisting of 700 stanzas, is an elaborate and insightful discourse on Yoga, and has been venerated by the Indian tradition as part of the *Vedic* (*Shruti* or 'revealed') literature. The *Bhagavad Gita* unfolds as a running dialogue in which Arjuna is instructed by Krishna on the exemplary way of living life wholly and meaningfully without getting 'stuck' in the thoughts of whatever gains or losses might accrue in the process. The Gita exposition is remarkably assimilative in that it seeks to reconcile the seemingly divergent philosophies of the *Vedas*, *Upanishads*, *Sankhya-Yoga*, and Brahmanism, not to speak of the devotional worship of a personal God in Krishna. As a treatise encompassing ethics, metaphysics and ontology in one sweep, the *Bhagavad Gita* delineates a three-fold path to salvation—*karma-yoga* (yoga of detached action), *jnana-yoga* (yoga of intellectual knowledge) and *bhakti-yoga* (yoga of devotion). Departing somewhat from the world negation implicit in the asceticism that finds favour with some Upanishads, the Gita expounds the ideal of detached action. Most favoured however, is the composite Yoga of devotion, surrender, meditation and mantra repetition as, with diligent practice, it is sure to expand the seeker and finally merge him in the ultimate reality—the all embracing Supreme Self of Krishna.

Patanjali: 300AD-400AD

It fell upon Patanjali's *Yoga Sutra* ('threads of yoga') to lend yoga its classical form as one of the six philosophical schools of Hindu Thought. From Patanjali onwards, yoga became an identifiable system rather than a loose conglomeration of amorphous spiritual speculations which underlay sundry observances. Patanjali probably lived around the 4th century AD although his dates and even his true identity are uncertain. A true adept of yoga both in theory and practice, he is popularly (but erroneously) believed to be the father of yoga. He nevertheless made probably the biggest impact on the development of yoga and his system, in due course, came to be known as Classical Yoga. The *Yoga Sutra* is a remarkably terse work—195 aphorisms arranged in four chapters describing ecstacy (*samadhi*), means of attainment (*sadhana*), paranormal powers (*vibhuti*) and isolation (*kaivalya*). The threads are intended as pointed allusions rather than elaboration on the structure and meaning of the yoga practices. They do not lend themselves to easy understanding or practice, and call for studied explanation so as to betray their true meaning and methods of practice.

It is the *Yoga Sutra* which gives us the *asthanga*, or eight-limbed *raja-yoga* that still forms bulk of the Classical Yoga curriculum. These eight steps, in hierarchical order are—

1. *Yama* — External restraints
2. *Niyama* — Internal observances
3. *Asana* — Postures
4. *Pranayama* — Breath control
5. *Pratyahara* — Sense withdrawal
6. *Dharana* — Concentration
7. *Dhyana* — Meditation
8. *Samadhi* — Ecstacy

Yama is a group of injunctions quite akin to the Ten Commandments. The injunctions comprise—(a) *ahimsa*—non-injury to any living being, (b) *satya*—truthfulness in thought and action, (c) *asteya*—nonstealing and noncovetousness, (d) *brahmacharya*—chastity and sublimation of sexual energy, and e) *aparigraha*—greedlessness. Likewise, *Niyama* consists of five practices—(a) *shaucha*-purity or cleanliness, (b) *santosha*—contentment, (c) *tapas*—asceticism, (d) *svadhyaya*—study and (e) *ishwar pranidhana*—surrender in Lord. The *Yama* and *Niyama* put together, foster high morals and have the right uplifting and purging influence on the mind, so as to make it fit for meditation.

Asana means a steady and comfortable posture with the trunk, neck and head held straight in an alignment so as to allow *prana*, the life energy, free flow along the bodily axis. In order to reach higher levels of mental concentration, one must be able to rise above body-consciousness. *Asanas* purify and strengthen the organs and the nervous system, and thereby facilitate mental concentration and flow of vital energy.

Pranayama is recognized as one of the principal means of revitalising the body and slowing down the ageing process. The higher purpose of *pranayama* however, is to control the incessant movement of the mind. Basically, it has three phases—(a) *puraka* or inhalation, (b) *kumbhaka* or retention and (c) *rechaka* or exhalation.

Pratyahara is essentially a fasting for the mind. The *Yoga Sutra* defines it as the simulation by the senses of the nature of consciousness, insofar as the senses sever themselves from their respective objects. This 'switching off' produces a state of introversion that is conducive to realisation of higher states. These five psychophysical steps then, form the basis for accomplishment of three remaining steps which are essentially spiritual.

Dharana is defined in the *Yoga Sutra* as the 'tethering of consciousness to a single locus'. It is therefore, the practice of *ekagrata* or one-pointedness of mind that comes with unwavering attention. The concentration-practice which is normally mistaken as meditation, is basic to the yoga process of introversion, aiding as it does a compacting of the psychospiritual energies. Objects of concentration can be anything ranging from a particular point in the space between the two eyebrows—the *nasikagra*—to an internalised image of the chosen deity.

Dhyana is defined as the unidirectional flow of impinging ideas with respect to a single object of concentration. Patanjali clarifies that any object that appeals to higher senses, can serve as an aid to meditation. Meditation leads to the arresting (*nirodha*) of the five kinds of fluctuations (*vritti)* of consciousness.

Samadhi, the final limb of *Patanjali-yoga* is that highest condition in which a complete merging of the subject and the object takes place. It is preceded by complete sense-withdrawal and highest meditation.

Post Patanjali

The *Yoga Upanishads* came after Patanjali and remained true to the *Upanishadic* tradition in that they still recognized an essential oneness underlying all existence: realizable through use of correct techniques of breathing and concentration that unleashed latent energies of sound and light. The *Yoga Upanishads* prepared the ground for a relatively more esoteric form of yoga practice, the *Kundalini-yoga*, that had been familiar to the adepts, but that increasingly came to the fore, involving the many. Techniques of directly accessing *prana* or the life-force from the physical body; stirring and raising it to the cerebral top in order to usher in the ecstatic state of unity, became central to the later *Yoga Upanishads.*

Tantricism: 100-600 AD

The origins of *Tantricism* are obscure, although the Tantra philosophy is widely believed to have arisen around the first century AD, and can be traced to a series of scriptural writings in Shaivism and even Buddhism. The cardinal concept in *Tantricism* is the idea of *Shakti,* the Goddess as the female principle of Cosmic Existence. The Tantra practitioner seeks to secure the awakening of this principle in the striving for Cosmic Union. This emphasis on the female cosmic principle necessitated a reassessment of the human anatomy and the physical aspect in general which had been of negative significance in the orthodox yoga traditions. Contrary to the ascetic systems of yoga, *Tantricism* upheld the body as the most useful instrument of Realization. At the same time, this reassessment of the body together with Shakti–oriented rituals, left space for occultism and allied practices. The great appeal of the Tantric path in the modern times nevertheless, stems from its overt acceptance of bodily pleasures.

Within *Tantricism,* two distinct approaches that evolved were (a) the *Dakshina marga,* or right hand path and (b) the

Vama marga, or the left hand path. The right hand path continued to employ more conservative means of achieving ecstatic unity, and was carried forward by the Shaivite sects using the *Siddha-yoga* methods of divine realization that are now familiar to the West. The more radical left hand path, which has earned *Tantricism* a bad name, attempted to reach ecstatic heights through a ritualistic use of the five infamous elements (*pancha-ma-kara*), specially sexual intercourse (*maithuna*).

It was the Tantra practitioners who first conceptualized specific models of the life-force inherent in the body, complete with its subtle energy vortices and the *Kundalini*-energy system that rises from the spinal base and terminates in the cerebral top. *Tantricism* also theorized on the importance of sound (*mantras),* hand postures aimed at retaining power (*mudras*) and precise, geometrical designs (*yantras*) to work at the energy vibrations. Even as the sexual rituals of *Tantricism* were explicit and unfettered, the partners were encouraged to rise above the revelling in transient, carnal pleasures of orgasm, aiming instead at the subtle energy streams for attainment of the ultimate bliss.

Hatha-yoga: 800–1700 AD

Hatha-yoga has continuously evolved from the times of *Goraksha*, a great medieval *Siddha* of the Natha tradition who lived around 10th century AD, and whose written works are now extinct. The *Hatha-Yoga-Pradipika* is the best known manual on *hatha-yoga,* written around 14th century. Describing *shatkarmas* (body cleansing methods), *pranayamas* (breath control techniques), *mudras* (energy retaining hand positions), and *asanas* (strongly held bodily postures) as significant yoga practices, it yet reconciles the physical aspects with the higher spiritual striving of *raja-yoga.*

Another work on *hatha-yoga* is the 17th century classic, the *Gheranda-Samhita.* This work, comprising 351 stanzas in seven chapters, is most significant for its enunciation of various forms of physical purification *(Shodhana)* meant for cleansing and massaging organs and internal passages. The *Gheranda-Samhita* mentions that there are all together 840,000 postures, out of which 84 are important for yoga practice.

Contemporary Yoga: 2000 AD

As already seen, *hatha-yoga* is only a fraction of Yoga, and yet has come to dominate yoga-practice in the modern times. Millions and millions of people outside India, are now practising yoga in some form or the other. The physical exercises of *hatha-yoga* have now increasingly become entwined with the psychospiritual disciplines of *raja-yoga* and *bhaktiyoga*. Most current yoga-practitioners look forward to yoga as the holistic key to longevity, cure, beauty and fitness. The specific yoga techniques have been found by medical research to be powerful therapeutic tools not only for promoting health and effecting cures, but also for slowing down the ageing and degenerative processes. Several 'involuntary' physiological processes such as heart rate and thyroid output that are vital parameters of health, have now been demonstrated by yoga adepts to be quite amenable to conscious control.

Yoga in the West: 1800—2000 AD

As noted earlier, Yoga at a theoretical level, was first introduced to the West in the 19th century by Swami Vivekananda, Ramkrishna's illustrious disciple. It was however, left to Paramahansa Yogananda in early 20th century, to inspire the Westerners on a large scale to understand and adopt *kriya-yoga*, an esoteric yoga variation making use of specific *asanas* and *pranayama* practices. Yogananda was the first adept yogi to stay in the Western countries over an extended period of time, and his famous *Autobiography of a Yogi* is a breath-taking, yet authentic tale of Yoga that deeply impacted Western sensibilities.

Another adept who helped establish yoga in the West, was Swami Sivananda. A fully illumined yoga-practitioner who was a qualified allopath physician to start with, he caused strong ripples in the nascent Western yoga-circles of the mid 20th century through his such noted disciples as Swami Vishnu Devananda (again a qualified allopath) and Swami Satyananda (whose Bihar School of Yoga at Munger, India attracts thousands of Westerners). Almost at the same time, Swami Muktananda, a great *Kundalini-yogi* of the *Shaivite Siddha-yoga* tradition, was also creating a deep impact in the West. His tradition of emphasizing *Shaktipat* initiation as the catalyst of yoga, is now being carried forward by his noted female disciple, Gurumayi Chidvilasananda, who is widely thought to be a *Siddha* herself.

At the turn of the new millennium, Yoga has become very much an important fabric of the Western cultures. Regrettably however, the yoga practitioners in the West have not always been well informed about the true dimensions of Yoga. Bereft of its spiritual context, yoga is now often practised in an alien hedonistic set up in much watered down, distorted versions that diminish its dignity and efficacy. In the event, it is pertinent to reflect whether the more esoteric and relatively purer forms of Yoga are relevant for the average Westerner. Orthodox yoga, specially one emphasizing *Kundalini*-energies and *Shaktipat,* is invariably triggered by a perfected master, or *Siddha* Guru. As I have strived to show however, the Westerner stands to equally benefit from even the most esoteric yoga traditions provided he is prepared to work that much harder in order to overcome the barriers of language, culture and ethnocentric values.

To Recap

1. The Vedas, arguably the oldest known scriptures in the history of mankind dating back to 4000 BC or

earlier, are the fountain-head of Yoga and all related Hindu metaphysics.

2. The Upanishads, comprising some 200 mystical writings and dated at around 1000 BC, are the next important landmark in the yoga history, emphasizing contemplation and meditation as major elements of yoga–practice and as means to Self–realization.
3. The *Mahabharata*, one of the two Epics that are the cornerstone of the Hindu way of life, was written around 100 AD, and is most famous for containing a rare yogic discourse in the form of the *Bhagavad Gita*.
4. With Patanjali's *Yoga Sutra*, Yoga becomes established in its classical, eight–limbed form as one of the six Hindu philosophical schools, and as an identifiable system.
5. The *Yoga Upanishads* came after Patanjali and remained true to the *Upanishadic* tradition in emphasizing the essential oneness of all existence realizable through techniques of breathing and concentration. It also prepared the ground for *Kundalini–yoga,* an esoteric form of yoga practice.
6. *Tantricism*, believed to have originated around 1st century AD, gained in prominence in the later *Upanishadic* period with its recognition of *Shakti*, the Goddess as the female cosmic principle, and with its overt acceptance of bodily pleasures.
7. With *Tantricism*, came the first specific models of the *Kundalini* energy system and the subtle energy centres, with attending emphasis on *mantras*, *mudras* and *yantras* as means to manipulating energy vibrations.
8. The two medieval classics that form the basis of *hatha-yoga* are the *Hatha–Yoga-Pradipika* and the *Gheranda-Samhita*, written between 14th and 17th century AD. Incorporating *asanas*, *pranayamas*,

mudras and *bandhas* as important yoga practices, *hatha-yoga* yet reconciles the physical aspects with the higher discipline of *raja-yoga.*

9. Contemporary yoga draws heavily from *hatha-yoga* and seeks to blend it with elements of *raja-yoga* and *bhakti-yoga* for promoting health, effecting cures and arresting degenerative processes.
10. Yoga was introduced to the West in 19th century by Vivekananda and was increasingly adopted by the westerners under the influence of Yogananda, then Sivananda and Muktananda.

IV. The Body

"Bernard (French Scientist) was right. The pathogen is nothing. The terrain is everything."

—Louis Pasteur (*shortly before his death*)

The Microcosm

To the positivists, objects are objective by virtue of their 'solidity'—their ability to be seen, felt and manipulated as also their amenability to precise laws of physics and mathematics. But exactly how is the flesh and blood of a famous movie actor any different from his walking image on the silver screen, is not that easy to answer. Granted, the image would only occupy two dimensions instead of the regular three, which implies that the 'real' stuff, as against the fake, would stand out as our senses of touch, sight and smell ventured closer. This approach nonetheless, however convincing and expedient at the level of common sense and everyday experience, shows serious limitations as we probe deeper. Much as we would like to wish that our sensory world was objective and real, science itself tells us that much like its image, the body of the movie actor was conjured up quite literally out of nothing. In the scientist's relentless search for the ultimate constituents of the human anatomy, organs stand reduced to tissues, tissues to cells, cells to molecules, molecules to atoms, atoms to protons/electrons, protons/electrons to quarks, and finally, on to nothing. Each of the atoms inside us is 99.999 percent empty space. Subatomic particles, the essential building blocks of matter, are not 'things' but interconnections between things. Again, these things are interconnections between other things....and so on ad infinitum. Modern science then, pictures matter not as solid and passive, but as continuously dancing and vibrating energy. Accordingly, our body is nothing but energy vibrating at a particular frequency. Rather than being a *thing*, it is a *process.* Beneath the body's chimera of shape and size, the reality is one of pure and 'permanent' change—we get a completely new skeleton every three months, a new skin every month and a new intestinal tract lining every day! And 80 percent of the liver when cut away, regenerates itself from the remains in a matter of hours! As we sift through this apparently solid body, we do not have to go too far before we are up against a fistful of 'nothing'. This *nothing* however, instead of being a void, is a throbbing inner space pregnant with thoughts, emotions and impressions that 'fill' life.

Not surprisingly then, scientists have described the human body, specially the brain, as the most complex structure in the known universe. The inconceivably complex structure, dynamics and functions of the tiniest parts of the human body continue to baffle and fascinate the greatest of scientific minds. The singular lack of success in comprehending one's own self, teeming with precision, intelligence and design, should in itself be reason enough to fill the thinking among us with awe and reverence for the Creator. Consider the vastness of this 'inner universe'. Close to 50 trillion cells or separate living entities inhabit this world, out of which about 100 millions are born and die every minute. An estimated 1 lakh chemical reactions take place in the brain every second. That no external toxins are needed to destroy the body and no external help suffices to save it in the unlikely event of the body's taken-for-granted inner Intelligence going wrong is best exemplified by the dreaded auto-immune disease of *myasthenia gravis* in which the body attacks its own cells. In this disease, the nerve/muscle junction appears like pathogenic bacteria to the circulating immune system cells, which attack the vital communication link between the neurological system and muscle function with usually fatal consequences.

The Cell

A cell is essentially a bag, wrapped in an outer membrane or the 'cell–wall', containing a blend of water and certain whirling chemicals. The 'nucleus' which forms the core of the cell, protects strands of DNA's bunched together. DNA—the fundamental chemical unit of life—tucked inside the cell, programmes it among other things, to split at a particular rate in order to produce two new cells. Far from being a 'mindless' mechanical process, cell–division is an extremely well coordinated, intelligent activity geared to meet its own internal needs and respond to chemical signals emanating from the surrounding cells, the brain and the organ–systems. How precise, intricate and sensitive the process of cell–division is, can be gauged from the fact that the tiniest aberration in this process results in the deadly disease of cancer. Inside the cell, each of our 30,000 genes is a specific instruction for life encoded in a precise sequence of four chemical letters—A, T, C and G—that would use up 750 megabytes of computer storage if represented as a string of letters. In an ascending order of palpability, cells come together to form tissues, tissues gather to make organs, organs give rise to systems and systems, to the human body, as we see it. At the other end, cells are themselves instructed by molecules or more specifically peptides, on when to divide, which protein to manufacture and which genes to activate. That these peptides themselves nearly miraculously spring from thoughts, thus enabling us to take a quantum leap from matter to mind, is something that we would dwell on later.

The Systems

Any description of the various parts of the human anatomy, and their functioning would generally include the following:

(i) *The five senses*

Comprised of the skin, eyes, nose, ears and tongue, they manipulate the external stimuli to let us feel the world outside.

(ii) *The endocrine system*

This comprises ductless glands that produce hormonal secretions passing directly into the blood stream. These are the pituitary, the thyroid, the parathyroid, the thymus, the adrenal, the reproductive and the pancreas. These glands are spread over the entire body and they have a decisive role in the playing out of our physiological and psychological states.

The *pituitary,* called the master gland for its regulatory action over all the other glands, lies between the eyes and in the rear of the nose. Among the many crucial functions of the pituitary is a life saving response to distress and emergency. The *thyroid* regulates growth, general metabolism and our mental well-being. The *parathyroid* ensures a balanced calcium and phosphorous ratio in the bones and blood. The *thymus* has a crucial bearing on the immune system through production of T-Lymphocytes. The adrenal glands are actually two; the *cortex* manufactures cortico-steroids that ensure the sodium–potassium balance, regulates the glucose level and controls production of sex hormones. The other adrenal gland—*medulla*—manufactures adrenaline that has the effect of raising blood sugar level and the blood pressure. Adrenaline secretion greatly increases in times of excitement, anger, fear, etc. The reproductive glands in woman are the *ovaries* that produce estrogen and progesterone, and control development of the female figure and reproduction. Testosterone, the male counterpart, holds the key to changes in voice, muscle building, reproduction and other male characteristics. Interestingly, ei-

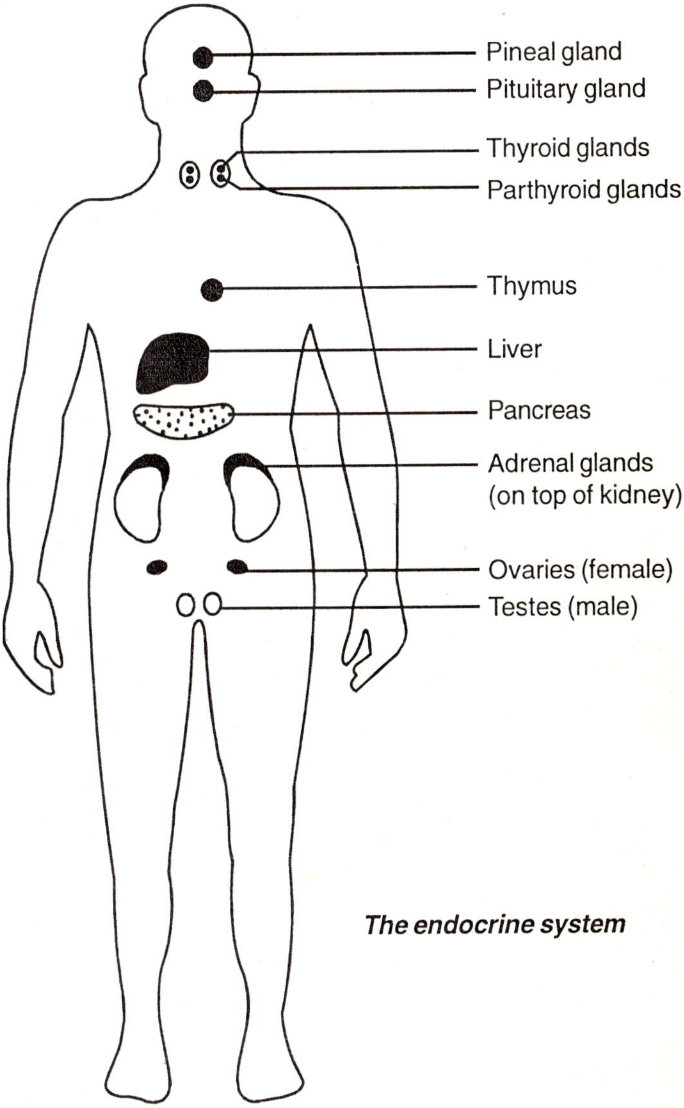

The endocrine system

ther sex produces small amounts of the opposite sex's hormones. Finally the *pancreas* produces insulin which controls blood sugar level and conversion of sugar into energy.

(iii) *The skeleton system*

This includes the ribs and skull that protect the softer organs and body tissues.

(iv) *The mascular system*

Contributing half of the total body weight, this renders possible both, our voluntary and involuntary movements.

(v) *The vascular system*

This includes the heart, blood–vessels, blood, lymphatic vessels and the lymph. At the core of the system is the *heart.* At birth, the heart beats at 130-160 times a minute, only to slow down with age to an average of just over 70. In a 24 hour cycle in an adult, it pumps 36,000 litres of blood that in turn traverses 20,000 kms of blood vessel length. Of the two systems of circulation, the *systemic* circulation takes the blood around the body, while the *pulmonary* circulation carries the blood to and from the lungs. The blood vessels that proceed from the heart and carry oxygenated blood, are known as *arteries.* The arteries are elastic, hollow and tapering as they spread through the body, with the smallest being known as capillaries. The blood vessels that take the de-oxygenated blood to the heart are called *veins.* Veins are elastic tubes equipped with valves to prevent back flow of the blood. The blood—five to six litres of them in the average adult—has four main components. These are *plasma, red corpuscles, white corpuscles* and *platelets.* Plasma is the liquid base of blood holding urea, sugar, mineral salts, enzymes and amino-acids in solution. Red corpuscles take their red colour from hemoglobin that can absorb oxygen. These cells take the oxygen around the body, and on the journey back carry waste products, specially carbon dioxide. White corpuscles are larger than the red ones and have a nucleus. They are manufactured in the bone marrow, and give protection from infection, multiplying rapidly in an emergency. Platelets, also generated in the bone marrow are vital for coagulation.

(vi) *The lymphatic system*

This is another circulatory system, interlinked with the blood circulation. *Lymph,* the liquid base, nourishes the tissue cells and expels waste.

(vii) *The nervous system*

Together with the endocrine glands, the nervous system controls the body through an efficient and coordinated system of exchange and operation. It is divided into two main parts—the central nervous system and the autonomic nervous system comprising the sympathetic and parasympathetic. All internal organs over which we have no control, have a dual nerve access to the *autonomic nervous system;* the *sympathetic* system increases body activity while the *parasympathetic* slows down the same.

The *brain,* encased in the protective skull, has 12 billion neurons or nerve cells. Its three main parts are—the cerebrum, the medulla oblongata and the cerebellum. The *cerebrum* forms bulk of the nervous system and comprises the right and left cerebral hemispheres. The two hemispheres are connected and constantly exchange information. For example, music is heard with the left hemisphere, but felt with the right side. The cerebrum has different areas controlling different functions. The *Frontal* lobe regulates intellect, reasoning and motor movement. The *Parietal* controls symbols and ideas, sensory taste and awareness. The *Occipital* is responsible for vision and discrimination. While the *Temporal* controls auditory function, language and speech. The brain's base, *medulla oblongata* connects the cerebellum and cerebrum to the spinal cord. It controls involuntary functions such as breathing, heart beat and digestion. The *cerebellum* mainly controls muscle coordination and body–equilibrium. The *spinal cord*, that is an extension of the medulla oblongata spans the vertebrae distributing the messages from the 'headquarters' to the entire body.

In the middle of the brain is the *thalamus* which acts as the central switching station for all sensory input, except smell. Beneath the thalamus is the tiny but functionally crucial *hypothalamus* that regulates body temperature, water metabolism, hunger, sleep, pleasure. Destruction of the hypothalamus leads to instant death.

(viii)*The digestive system*

It processes and converts the food intake into usable fuel for energy, growth and repair. The digestive tract begins at the mouth and finishes at the anus. From the mouth where it is partially broken down by the saliva, the food passes via the pharynx and the esophagus into the stomach. The stomach has glands manufacturing gastric juice that contains the enzymes, pepsin and rennin, and hydrochloric acid. The food then passes into the *small intestine*, and on into the larger intestine, with its useful content absorbed, and the residual waste eventually being evacuated through the anus.

The digestive system is aided by the liver and the pancreas. Liver, the largest organ in the body, has several functions, the most important being to produce and store bile. Bile passes to the *gall bladder*, to get concentrated many times over and stored until required, when it passes into the *duodenum,* that is the first part of the small intestine. Bile contains salts and pigments got from the disintegrated red blood cells. Bile salts are reabsorbed to promote efficient digestion of fat.

(ix) *Respiratory system :*

It takes oxygen into our bodies and ejects carbon dioxide and water. Lungs, located inside the rib cage, are the chief organ of the respiratory system. Through contraction and relaxation of the muscular wall, called *diaphragm*, the atmospheric air is sucked in and ejected alternately to cause breathing. Fresh air is ingested and its oxygen off-loaded to the blood in return for the disposable carbon dioxide for the next breath to come and expel the waste.

(x) *Genito-urinary system :*

It comprises the excretory and the reproductive organs with overlapping functions. The chief organs are the female specific *ovaries, fallopian tubes* and *uterus* along with the gender common *urethra* and the *urinary bladder*. The urinary part includes the *kidneys* whose function it is to segregate certain waste products from the blood so as to ensure maintenance of a constant composition of the blood despite variations in type and amount of dietary and fluid intake. Around 150 litres of fluid are processed by the kidney in 24 hours, but only 1 percent of it leaves as urine.

The above then is a rough approximation of what the vastly complex human body is like inside out. A more exhaustive account of its interior is neither possible nor desirable in a work of this nature which sees the physical frame as a vehicle for the transcendental influences of the spirit, rather than as life's *raison d'etre.*

Manna from heaven

A few more words about the working of the endocrine system however, seem to be in order. True to the then prevailing isolationist mood in the medical science of the 70's and before, a majority of researchers were convinced that each gland and organ system functioned singly and independently to the exclusion of all other glands and organ systems. Gradually it was found out that the endocrine glands function holistically; closely interacting and coordinating with all other glands and cells of the immune system. Evidence then started to trickle in, of the existence of a certain governing agency in the body that was geared to facilitate and synchronize the exchange of information and to dispense all the related functions. This governing agency, it now turns out, is the *pineal gland.* Till recently ignored as "useless" by the medical science, this pea-sized gland, located at the brain's centre, has now come to be viewed as the "super master" gland on account of its close proximity to, and decisive influence on the functioning of the pituitary. *Pinoline*, a beta-carboline suspected to have a major role in clairvoyance, extrasensory perception and out-of-body experience, is secreted by the pineal.

The *pineal* is also the body's ageing clock that regulates the ageing process through secretion of the magic hormone, *melatonin.* Melatonin in turn, sends information to all other systems in the body on the manner, timing and pace of ageing. Our physical body grows up, matures and degenerates the way it does because the melatonin level in the pineal gland programmes it to do so. In an adult body, the melatonin flow peaks at around the age of twenty and is halved by the time we reach sixty. Beyond the age of sixty, the melatonin level dips sharply as we approach the twilight. We can trust our immune system to be bouncy and firm so long as the pineal discharges enough of melatonin, vivifying and shielding us with high lymphocyte counts to produce antibodies and banish toxic invaders. A high level of melatonin also ensures a high thyroid output keeping our energy levels high. Really, for the body under siege from such enemies as ageing, stress and infection, melatonin is *manna from heaven.*

The Defences

If the inner structures of the body are ingenious, then its defences are no less fascinating, programmed as they are to screen, eject or exterminate a variety of potentially deadly invaders. The skin is the first line of defence. Silently but surely, it is all the time stopping a host of enemies—virus, bacteria, parasites and fungi—from sneaking in. Then comes a whole battery of first line defences designed to ward off invasions and stop micro-organisms from entering the blood This comprises a set of barriers including:

- the mucus membranes in the mouth, nose, ears etc.
- tears in the eyes
- the acid pH balance
- the acid juices that destroy anything that is able to make it as far as the stomach

Lysozyme is found in tears, sweat, saliva and urine. This enzyme works by breaking down bacterial cell walls. Beyond this first line defence, the formidable internal security of the immune system takes over. Specialized white blood cells trigger the production of antibodies and other agents in order to stop the spread of infection. Among the most important of these is *interferon,* which acts as a messenger, crossing over from infected cells to adjacent healthy cells, forewarning and equipping them.

Intriguingly, the body cells that were earlier seen to individually carry a complete blue print of the entire body including their own, also possess a gate pass with which to be whisked in. Cells known as *lymphocytes*, as soon as they detect trespassers, produce a protein molecule. This *antibody* is so manufactured as to neatly sit on the surface of the invader or *antigen* like a lid. If the reassuring presence of one such antibody is music to the ears, consider this—one single drop of blood may contain trillions of such antibodies! When an antibody is up against the antigen, one of several things may happen. The antibody can incapacitate the enemy on its own. Else it can cling on to the enemy and aid special fighter cells in finishing them off. Lastly, it can dent the intruder for other molecules to move in for the kill. White blood cells trained in the thymus gland to engage invaders and destroy them are known as T-cells. The trillions of white blood cells have the ability to recognize the intruder, recall how they were handled before and retaliate.

Disease

The impressive march past of the defence army might make us wonder as to how in spite of all this arsenal, man still finds himself often at the receiving end of a whole range of dreaded diseases. It may therefore, be pertinent to note that much as our bodies are armoured and equipped, they have to contend with the trickiest of adversaries. A *virus*, that most slippery of customers, is usually the width of twenty to hundred nanometers (1 nanometer = 1 millionth of a millimeter). It is actually a bunch of DNA's or RNA's wrapped inside a protein envelope that is ever on the lookout for a host cell. Once the virus infiltrates a host cell, the protective envelope is torn open and ingeniously, the virus uses the host cell to replicate itself. All this conspiring goes on inside the cell, so the virus is safe from most of the body's defences. In order to tackle them, the body ought to have special defences. This special defence, as seen, comes in the form of white cells that swing into action the moment they receive distress signals from the infiltrated cell. Interferon causes cells to manufacture other proteins that inhibit the proliferation of the virus.

Drugs, so effective against the bacteria have so far remained largely ineffectual against the marauding virus. Our body is, therefore, as yet, the best defence in its own battle of attrition against the virus. That our own inner environment may hold the key to end the virus menace, is indicated by new research centred on the use of "good" bacteria to control injurious viral activity. Special strains of specific bacteria, especially the *lactobacilli*, have been seen to secrete vivacidal compounds that actually kill viruses. Dr. Metchnikoff, a Nobel Prize winner, discovered why the yogurt-loving Bulgarians lived significantly longer than the rest. It was all thanks to the friendly bacteria contained in yogurt, which Dr. Metchnikoff named *Lactobacillus Bulgaricus*.

Neuro-peptides

In the last quarter of the 20th century, there came into reckoning a totally new genre of micro-chemicals—the neuro-peptides that are now viewed as the first physical manifestation of thought. The neuro-peptides were the first major step forward in bridging the gulf between the dynamic and ever-mutating realities of mind and body. Brain researchers, through a process known as *positron—emission tomography*, were now able to photograph a thought's tracks in 3–D. Research showed that each specific mental event triggers a distinct chemical pattern in the brain and by extension, that *each thought, in effect, rearranges the whole body*. At any given time therefore, *our body is but a 3-D picture of our thoughts!* It also turned out that the commonsensical tendency to look at biochemicals such as neurotransmitters and the DNA as belonging to the body rather than the mind, was expedient, but unsatisfactory. For, DNA's—all 3 billions of them—are palpable matter at one extreme and, pure knowledge at the other. Similarly, a cell was best conceived as a memory that had gathered some matter around itself to form a particular pattern. The convenient functional division of the body into the endocrine, the neurological, the vascular and such other systems, increasingly became discredited as scientists realized that everything is fused and synergized at the level of the neuropeptide.

Just as in quantum physics light behaves now as a wave, now as a particle, in new biology, the same mind–body event is seen to manifest now as a thought, now as a neuro-peptide. And just as light cannot be a wave and a particle at the same time, the mind–body event cannot be a thought and a neuro-peptide at the same time. As the DNA is divided and sub-divided into atoms and sub-atomic particles, we are left with nothing unless we conceive of some quantum construct that underlies both energy and matter, the thought and the neuro-peptide. For want of a better word, this quantum construct can be simply described as intelligence. Intelligence then, can assume the form of a thought, or a molecule—more specifically, a neuro-peptide. The greater challenge before science in the 21st century, one suspects, is going to be that of probing and demystifying laws of the inner space, rather than of the outer, in which new medicine and biology are likely to emulate the new physics. The first signs of quantum biology being born at the turn of the new millennium have come in the form of cracking of the human genome, deciphering the genetic text from the raw DNA mass.

The Genome "Spell-Check"

In less than one-and-a-half decade, some of the finest scientific minds have come together to unmask the blueprint of life that humans only speculated about for close to 5,000 years of civilized life. Quite startlingly, as against conventionally accepted and a rather flattering figure of one lakh that has turned out to be way off the mark, we are now seen to have only 30,000 genes—about the same as mice, twice as many as the round-worm and only five times more than the bacteria. Diseases, it now turns out, are just "spelling mistakes" in a normal gene. The Human Genome Project gives scientists an instant spell-check and the tools to correct the defects. Designer drugs, predictive medicine and "doctored" or "engineered" genes "to end the disease menace" now seem to be round the corner. Are we then at the mind-boggling threshold of producing supermen and playing God? Not quite, as Genome scientists are the first to concede.

Till recently, scientists were smug in the belief that once the human genome was mapped out, identifying each gene responsible for each human function would be easy. There was a genome, say, for cancer, asthma, alcoholism, diabetes, depression, schizophrenia and so on; prevention/cure was just a matter of 'tailoring' this or that 'culprit' gene. Fortunately or unfortunately, this cocky optimism has just been shown the door. Among the many startling findings of the ambitious and much talked about Human Genome Project, the one that is perhaps the most significant is that genes function in a context and more like networks than as single entities breeding specific proteins. This could be the key to understanding why despite the relatively low gene-count in humans, they are a much more complex and sophisticated life form than the lowly mice that has about the same number and kind of genes. Over and above this far more holistic and creative model of the genome is the surfacing of things that refuse to fit the jigsaw. Genes by themselves, for example, occupy only 1.5 percent of chromosomal space—the rest having so far been viewed dismissively as 'junk'. Scientists are now inclined to give a long and hard new look at this 'junk' that could really hold the key to unravelling the great secrets of evolution. In this sense, the real journey in self–discovery may have just begun rather than ended.

The purpose of writing so extensively on the physical body and the biochemical processes involved, that might seem odd in a essentially spiritually oriented work, is not to overwhelm the laid back reader with technical jargon, or drown him in scientific details. It is rather to convince the most scientifically inclined among the yoga seekers, of the all-pervasive nature of the ever happening yoga in their own flesh and blood quite unknown to them. To those who have a first impression of yoga and meditation as something distant, hollow and elusive, it might yet dawn that, unknown to them, each drop of their blood, each fibre of their flesh, each burst of melatonin, each trickle of interferon, each neuro-peptide, each DNA is being guided every moment by a Supreme Intelligence to silently and ceaselessly do Yoga in the master's cause. If we still do not give yoga its due and join in, the choice is ours, till compulsion comes in the form of a ravaged body, an unstable mind, and a warped spirit.

To Recap

1. Scientists know the human brain to be the most complex structure in the known universe.
2. Human body, far from being solid, is composed almost entirely of 'nothing'. It is actually a 3-D picture of our thoughts.
3. Rather than being a receptacle, the body is actually a flow; we get a new skeleton every three months and a new skin in one month.
4. The key systems of the body—the endocrine, the skeletal, the vascular, the neurological, the digestive, the respiratory and the genito-urinary—function with a precision and ingenuity that is difficult to explain without an underlying Intelligence.
5. The pineal gland, located at the cerebral top and now recognized as the governing agency of the body, is the ageing clock that secretes the magic hormone *melatonin*, and subtly occasions bodily changes.

6. The pineal secretions are also suspected to have a role in 'supernormal' experiences.
7. The best doctor that the body can have is the body itself, by way of its intricate and seemingly impregnable defences.
8. Disease still occurs because the foreign invaders, specially the virus, are equally cunning and surreptitious.
9. In the mind–body continuum, neuro-peptides are the mystery molecules that spring from thoughts and help build bridges between mind and matter.

V. The "Bodies"

"Whenever there is any manifestation of what is ordinarily called supernatural power or wisdom, there must have been a little current of Kundalini, which found its way into the susumna."

—SWAMI VIVEKANANDA

A strange thing happened in 1898. A full 14 years *before* the 'unsinkable' Titanic met its watery grave, Morgan Robertson published a weird novel '*The Wreck of The Titan*'. The novel foretold the Titanic disaster in such graphic detail and with such stunning accuracy, as was impossible without an actual vision of the tragedy that was to take place a decade–and–half later. Apart from the obvious similarity in names, both ocean liners—the fictional and the actual—were carrying over 2000 passengers and 20–odd life boats. Both were hit by icebergs at around the same speed of .24 knots. Both were 800 feet long or thereabouts, both had a displacement of around 70,000 tonnes, and finally, both sank in the North Atlantic ocean in the night of April. This, together with several well–recorded instances of *deja vu,* did much to lend credence to the emerging view that human consciousness, at times, functions independent of the physical body and finite intelligence, and that in doing so, it transcends the barriers of time and space.

Not many people are aware that death—cessation of the physical body—has been extensively and systematically researched in the last century by scientists working in the fields of parapsychology and psycho-kinesis. Some consciousness researchers, almost apologetically, are even coming round to conjecturing the existence of a human spirit. Latest findings in ESP and bio-electricity have been largely supportive of the yoga model of human body as an intricate hierarchic system of conjoined 'sheaths', or *koshas*, each oscillating at a different frequency and having its own degree of coarseness, rather the lack of it. Scientists have employed kirlian photography to detect a measurable field of bio-electricity around all animate entities. Quite remarkably, this bio-electric field around living things has been shown to survive their physical death for several hours. Research in the Chinese healing techniques of *acupressure* and *acupuncture* has also found tangible evidence of 'energy centres', bio-electric currents and 'meridians' that cannot be wished away by modern medicine. Of particular interest are *out of body experiences*(*OBEs*) that have been well documented over the years. There is substantial evidence that *OBEs* are more frequent than one might feel comfortable with, and that consciousness survives the physical body. Increasingly, it is being realized that the reporting of *OBEs* is often suppressed due to social inhibitions and the pressure to conform. Several authors, including such respectable names as William Wordsworth, Tennyson, D. H Lawrence and Virginia Woolf, have all described their own *OBEs* in no uncertain terms. And words such as *aura, kirlian photography, chakras and astral body* have become quite commonplace in Western yoga circles. There is enough reason to suspect that, just as the 20th century saw the revolutionary rise of quantum physics at the expense of its Newtonian cousin, the 21st century is poised to witness a decisive emergence of quantum medicine from the shadows of medical orthodoxy. For, the yoga model of human "bodies" doubtless scores over the purely physical allopathic model of human anatomy in explaining the recent findings of consciousness researchers. And equally significantly, it is much more in tune with contemporary physics as compared to 20th century medicine. Already, there are signs of allopathy coming to terms with the 'spirits'.

Researchers such as Richard Gerber, MD talk of the etheric body as a physical—etheric interface or ".... holographic energy template associated with the physical body".... and acknowledge that *"within the etheric energic map is carried information which guides the cellular growth of the physical structure of the body.... also the structural data for growth and repair of the adult organism, should damage or disease occur."*

Koshas

In *Taittiriya Upanishad*, our physical body is said to be but one tier of a system of five conjoined *bodies*. Accordingly, all human beings extend outward into the universe in five tiers or *koshas*. Beginning with the gross body of our everyday experience, these *koshas* are neatly arranged in the form of invisible sheaths in the following descending order of 'density':

(a) The *Annamaya Kosha*—the sheath composed of food
(b) The *Pranamaya Kosha*—the sheath composed of life-force
(c) The *Manomaya Kosha*—the sheath composed of mind
(d) The *Vijnanamaya Kosha*—the sheath composed of awareness
(e) The *Anandamaya Kosha*—the sheath composed of bliss

The yoga tradition also recognizes these human bodies more or less in the same terms, with slight variations in gradation and nomenclature. This roughly corresponds with the aura of Western occultism that signifies the subtle energy field enveloping the gross body. The distinct layers of the auric energy field—invisible to us, but easily seen by a *Siddha*—can be equated with different *koshas* of the yoga tradition. The aura photographed through the kirlian technique is the densest of the energy bodies—the etheric body—and can be equated with the *pranamaya kosha*. At a subtler level, the emotional aura or astral body corresponds with the *manomaya kosha*. A still subtler auric field corresponds with the *vijnanamaya kosha* or the causal body. Finally, there is the subtlest of all fields viz., the *anandamaya kosha* or the supracausal body, that is generally equated with the Supreme Self.

Nadis

According to the yoga texts, there are 720 million *nadis* or astral nerve-tubes in the human form that set the flow patterns of the psychosomatic energy. There is some debate specially in the West's interpretation of yoga as to whether the *nadis* should be regarded as physical or ethereal entities. The uncertainty stems largely from the fact that the *nadis* are said to perform different functions that lie in the grey zones between the material and the astral. For example, the *nadis* are said to be channels for blood on the one hand, and for *prana*, the life energy, on the other. In any case as Christopher Isherwood so pointedly observes in his biography of Ramakrishna, the Hindu philosophical system has always made light of the supposedly unbridgeable chasm between matter and energy, viewing them instead, as ever mutating aspects of the same fundamental Reality. That contemporary physics itself pictures matter as 'dancing energy' means that there is now hardly any room left for speculation or debate on this issue.

Among the 720 million *nadis* that constitute the human form, the three most important are the central conduit called the *susumna* along with two others that wind around it in helical fashion—the *ida* and the *pingala*. *Susumna* is the astral counter-part of the spinal cord, while the *ida* and *pingala* correspond respectively to the parasympathetic and sympathetic cords in the physical body. *Ida* is often called the 'moon' channel. Situated to the left of the susumna, it winds its way up from the bottom left side of the spine to the right nostril. *Pingala* is also known as the 'solar' channel. Situated to the right of the susumna, it begins its spiral upward rise from the bottom right side of the spine to the left nostril. *Ida* is a channel of cold or negative energy current, and *pingala* is the carrier of hot or positive energy currents. *Ida* and *pingala* are active in all human beings, since the breath comes in and goes out through these very *nadis*. In most people however, the *susumna nadi* is closed and remains unknown.

The axial channel of the *susumna*, nonetheless, is the most important of the 720 million *nadis*. Located between the *ida* and the *pingala* close to the spinal column, it is the central channel through which the life energy or *prana* can flow from the psycho-energetic centres or *chakras* at the spinal base to the cerebral top that houses the 'crown' centre. The *susumna* controls and regulates all other *nadis*, and through them, all the multifarious activities of human life. It extends in an unbroken, spiral line from the bottom of the spine—seat of the *muladhara* or the root *chakra*—to the cerebral-top centre, or the *sahasrara*.

Chakras

The *chakras* are to be found where the *ida* and the *pingala* cross. The *ida* and the *pingala* rise in the base chakra and terminate in the sixth chakra. The male and female principles, *Shiva* and *Shakti*, are internalized in the human body and occupy either end of the *susumna*. So long as the masculine and feminine, static and dynamic energies are divided, the human condition is not 'whole'. *Chakras* or the "wheels of fire" are the seven subtle energy centres located along the spine that form an integral part of the nerve plexuses. Graphically depicted as 'lotuses', they are junction points located one atop another along the *susumna* through which *Shakti* has to eventually pass on her way up to reunion with *Shiva.* Each *chakra* signifies a particular crisis that must be overcome. Each chakra is also a converging point of psycho-spiritual energies that must be kindled for the unfolding yoga process to run its full course. At the practical level, our psychological and spiritual impulses activate, and in turn are activated by, specific *chakras*. People 'bound' to the lower *chakras* are likely to gravitate towards relentless gratification of the physical senses. While those in touch with the higher *chakras* engage themselves in subtler pursuits involving fine arts, intellect and the spirit. All of us nonetheless, are attuned in varying degrees to a combination of *chakras*, engendering our abilities, attitudes and inclinations that are uniquely our own. At the same time, the higher *chakras* may be construed as stepping stones to the advanced yogic states that carry 'supernormal' abilities, or *siddhis* such as clairvoyance, clairaudience and healing in their wake.

Each *chakra* is depicted as a lotus with a fixed number of petals. The number of petals represents the number and position of *nadis* that branch out from the particular *chakra*. When the *Shakti* lies dormant, the *nadis* droop and face downward, only to turn around and 'blossom' lotus-like after awakening. Each petal is identified with one of the fifty Sanskrit sounds or letters, that represents the particular vibration produced on it by the *Kundalini-shakti* as it passes through the *chakra*. Over and above petals and sounds, each *chakra* possesses its own fixed geometric form, colour, element and presiding deity. The seven *chakras* may be briefly described as under:

(i) *Muladhara*—the 'Survival' chakra

The lowest of the *chakras*, this ' root' centre is located at the base of the spine, and is associated with the adrenal glands of the physical body. It is associated with the sense of smell, the element of earth, and the seed mantra or unmanifest sound of *'lam'*. The four crimson petals in clockwise order are associated with four different vibrations. The *Kundalini* lies dormant in three-and-half coils within this *chakra*. The presiding deity is Brahma and His consort, Dakini. The first of the three knots, or the *Brahmagranthi* (a *granthi* is a deadlock to be necessarily broken through with the aid of *yoga-sadhana* for the *Kundalini* to rise) is also located here. Meditation on this *chakra* brings control over breath and mind. It also brings the 'supernormal' ability to jump like a frog and, ultimately, to actually levitate.

(ii) *Svadhisthana*—the 'Pleasure' chakra

This 'self-base' centre, with six petals, is situated near the reproductive organ, and is related to the gonads—the ovaries, testicles and the prostrate gland. It is associated with the element of water, the sense of taste and the seed sound of '*vam*'. The six vermilion petals are represented by six different sounds. *Vishnu* and *Rakini* are the presiding deities. Meditation on this *chakra* brings intuition, psychic powers and access to astral beings. Interestingly, it is said to make the practitioner physically attractive specially to the opposite sex; a feat that can become a major test for the *sadhaka.*

(iii) *Manipura*—the 'Power' chakra

This centre 'shining like a pearl' with ten petals, is located near the navel at the solar plexus, and is related to the pancreas. It is associated with the element of fire, the sense of sight and with *bija mantra*, '*ram*'. The ten petals the colour of rain-clouds, are represented by ten different sounds. Presiding deities are *Rudra* and *Lakini*. Meditation on this *chakra* reveals secrets of medicinal remedies and brings exemption from fear of fire and disease. Significantly, it also enables the practitioner to leave his body at will and enter another.

(iv) *Anahata*—the 'Love' chakra

Also known as the heart centre, this centre of the '*unstruck* sound' is a twelve petalled *chakra* located in the region of the heart. The gland that it relates to is the thymus. This chakra is associated with the element of air, the sense of touch and the seed sound '*yam*'. The twelve deep red petals are associated with twelve Sanskrit sounds. Presiding deities are *Isha* and *Kakini.* The primal 'unstruck' sound of '*Shabda Brahma'* that comes without the beating of any two things together, is to be found here. Also, the second of the three knots, or the *Vishnu-granthi* is located here. Meditation on this *chakra* brings purity, universal love and higher psychic abilities.

(v) *Visuddha*—the Chakra of 'Miracles'

This '*pure*' centre, comprising 16 petals is located close to the throat, and is related to the thyroid. The element of ether, the sense of hearing and the sound of '*ham*' are associated with it. The 16 smoky purple petals have 16 different Sanskrit sounds. Presiding deities are *Sadasiva* and *Shakini.* Meditation on this *chakra* brings purification of intelligence and reveals knowledge of four Vedas. It also brings such paranormal abilities as clairvoyance and clairaudience.

(vi) *Ajna*—the 'Third Eye' chakra

Located at the '*third eye*'centre, between the two eyebrows, this 'command' centre has only two white petals and is associated with the pituitary. It is connected with the sense of individuality, or *ahamkara* and the seed letter '*Om*'. Presiding deities are *Parama Shiva* and *Devi Hakini.* Meditation on this *chakra* destroys karmas, and brings all paranormal abilities including telephathic communication and thought manifesting matter. *Siddhas* consciously put their *prana* into this *chakra* at the time of their physical death. This chakra is named as such because it acts as the receiver for the Guru's telepathic instructions to the worthy disciple. The last of the three knots, the *Rudra-granthi* is also located

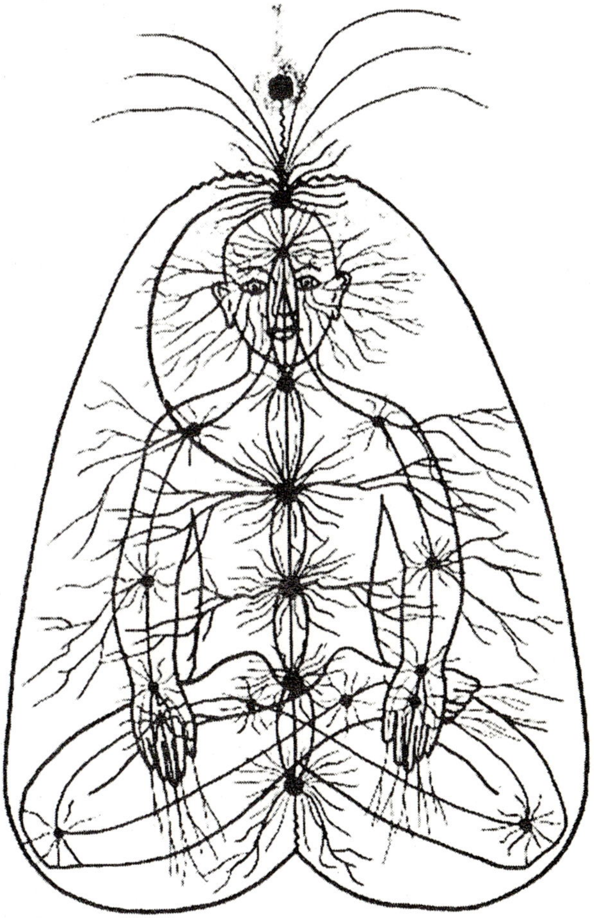

The network of astral nerve-tubes in the human 'bodies'.

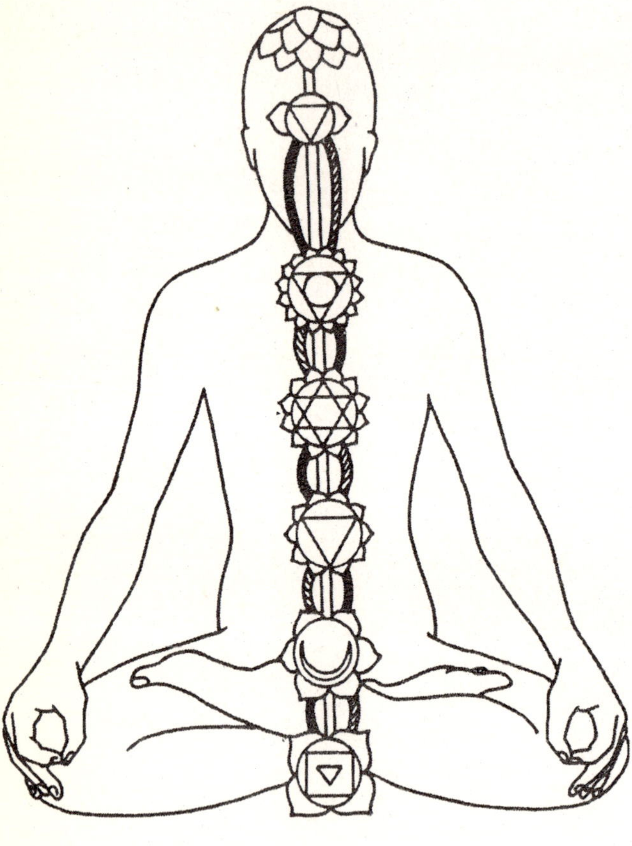

The subtle body with the seven Chakras

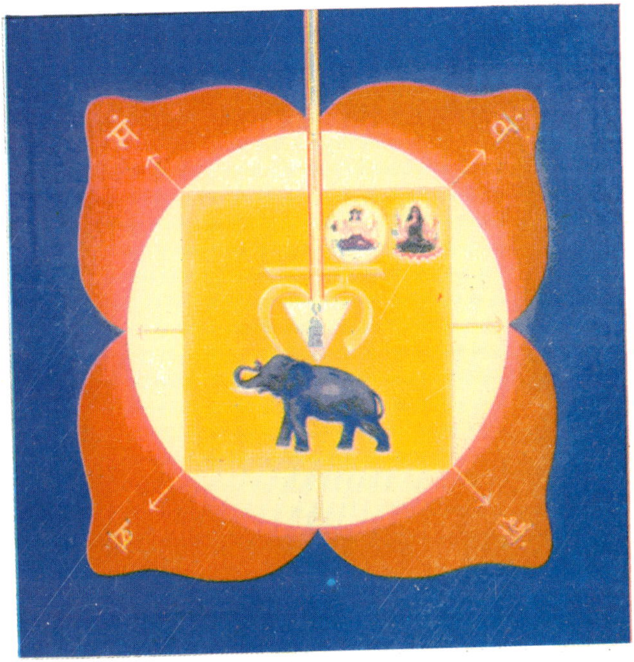

Mūlādhāra Chakra

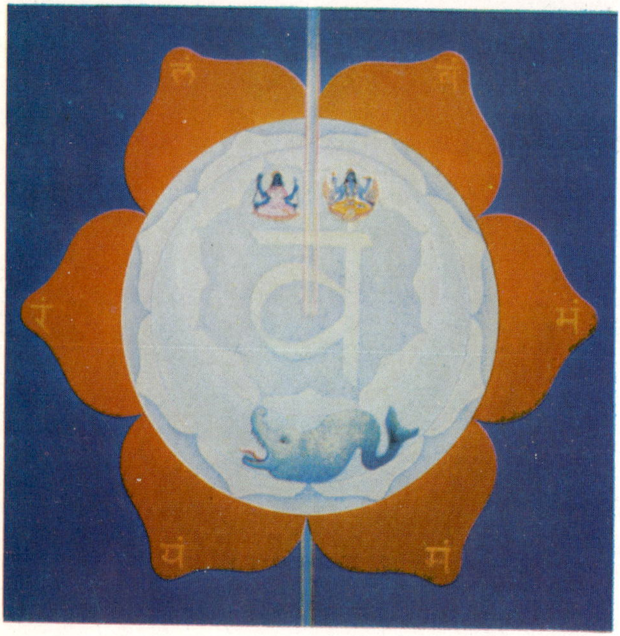

Svādhiṣṭhāna Chakra

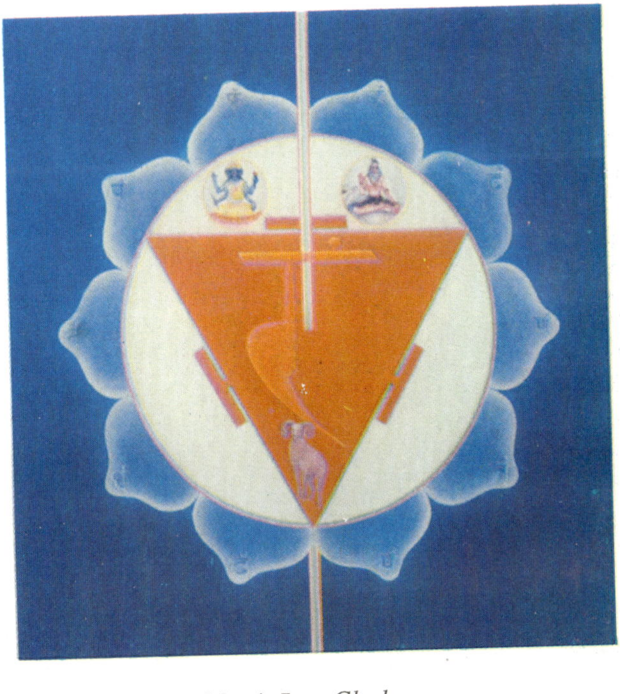

Maṇipūra Chakra

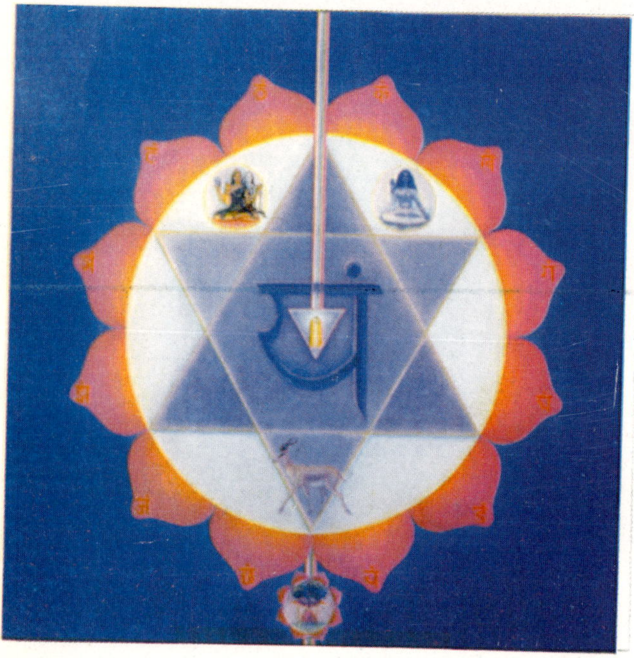

Anāhata Chakra

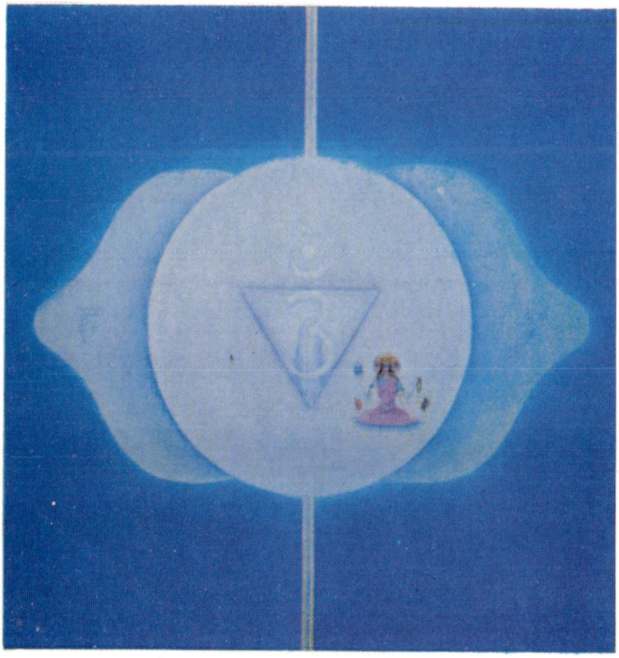

Ājñā Chakra

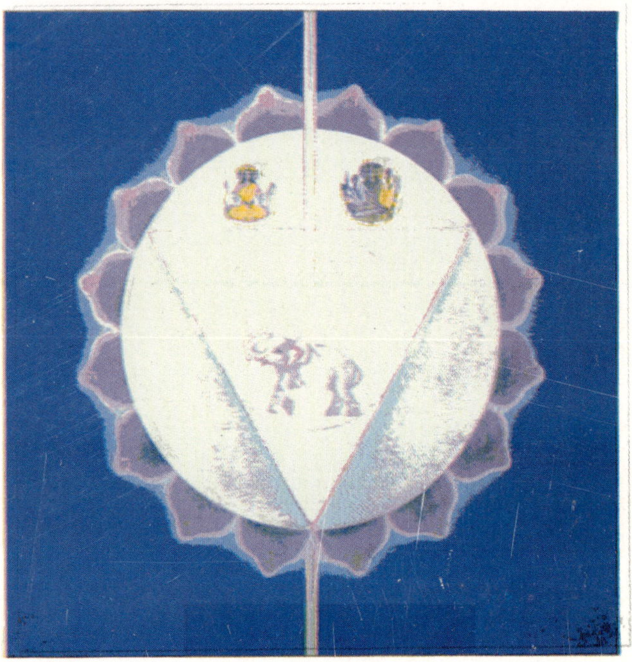

Viśuddha Chakra

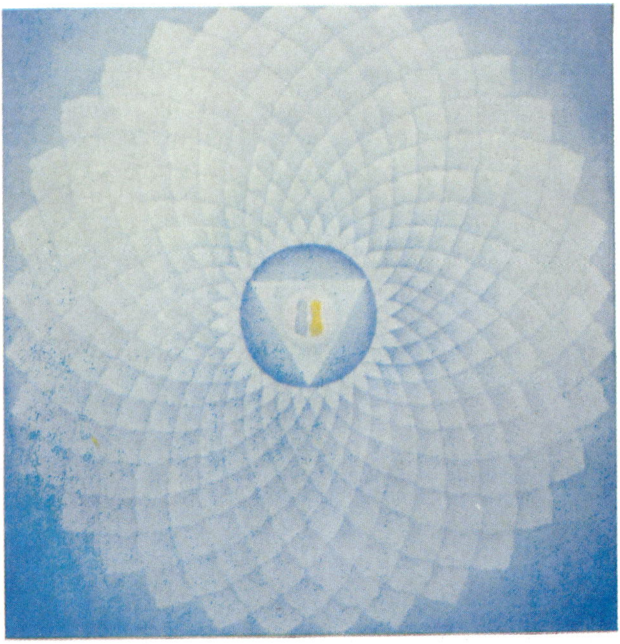

Sahasrāra

here.

(vii) Sahasrara—the 'Crown' chakra

This '*thousand petalled*' centre is located in the crown of the head, and is associated with the pineal gland. The thousand petals are arranged in twenty layers with all fifty Sanskrit sounds repeated on each. It is presided over by only one deity, Brahma, since all duality ceases here with the complete union of *Shiva* and the *Shakti* in the *Samadhi* state. When the physical end approaches, the *Siddha* cuts himself off from the mortal frame for the *sahasrara* centre to burst open, thus letting the *prana* escape.

ILLUSTRATION

Chakra	**Gland**	**Body-parts**	**Functions**
1. *Muladhara*	Adrenal	Spinal column	Survival, Procreation
2. *Svadhisthana*	Prostrate	Reproductive organs, Kidneys	Health, Pleasure
3. *Manipura*	Pancreas	Stomach, Gall bladder, Liver, Spleen	Energy
4. *Anahata*	Thymus	Heart, Lungs	Immune System
5. *Visuddha*	Thyroid	Throat, Bronchial tubes	Growth, Communication, Creativity
6. *Ajna*	Pituitary	Central Nervous System	Higher mind
7. *Sahasrara*	Pineal	Cerebrum	Human perfection

Prana

Prana is the vibrant psychophysical energy, the universal life force that finds mention in the oldest scriptures. In the *Rig Veda*, it signifies the breath of the Cosmic *Purusha.* The highly concentrated impact of *prana* unleashes the *Kundalini-shakti* and pushes it up the central channel in the yogi's journey to perfection. *Prana* and *apana* also signify inhalation and exhalation respectively. As such, in its internal aspect, *prana* also means the life force that enlivens the human being. In *Yoga Vasishtha*, it is defined as the vibrating power (*spandana Shakti*) that is the substratum of all phenomena.

Prana, known as *chi* in the Chinese system and as *ki* in the Japanese system, is the basis of oriental medicine. It is the *prana* that makes all our body systems and organs function. Physical illnesses stem from a basic disturbance in the energy pathways that impedes free flow of pranic energy. A copious and unhindered flow of *prana* is the key to all healing. Unlike the allopathic system, the yoga theory rather than viewing diseases as locally and externally caused, looks at them in terms of a fundamental imbalance of *prana.*

In the normal course, *prana* flows in the *ida* and *pingala* astral nerve tubes in a random, diffused manner. Systematic yoga practice however, enables the practitioner to tap much higher levels of the *pranic* energy allowing it to flow in the central channel of *susumna*, and thus activate the *chakra* in the form of *Kundalini* energy.

Kundalini

Kundalini is perhaps the least appreciated aspect of the Hindu thought, yet a concept of cardinal importance in yoga theory. In the New Age yoga–cult, when most metaphysical concepts such as karma, reincarnation, biofeedback, past life regression and astral travel are openly being bandied about, the most important of them, *Kundalini*, has largely remained at the fringes of yoga teachings and practice. Notwithstanding a few authentic accounts, such as '*The Serpent Power*' by Sir John Woodroffe, and the more recent writings of Gene Kieffer, the *Kundalini* research has largely remained in the margins. Most New Age yoga-gurus have preferred to remain reticent on the subject, probably because, given their lack of experience of the *Kundalini* working, they would otherwise be walking on very thin ice. Yet the *Kundalini* is a fact of life not only to the great *Siddhas*, but also to the common man. A proper theoretical grounding in the *Kundalini* is, therefore, of as much relevance to the yoga part-timer as for the yogis in the making.

Kundalini in one form or the other, finds mention in nearly all traditions. Maya and ancient Egyptians knew it. So did the Greeks, the Tibetans and the Sufis. As mentioned, the Chinese know this primal energy as '*Chi*' or '*Qi*', the Japanese as '*Ki*', and the Bible calls it the '*Holy Spirit*'. In the spiritual traditions of the African aborigines, *Kundalini* is accepted as the sacred energy that restores man to his divine essence. The Native Americans have this conviction that man and the 'living earth' were constructed alike—a belief that has shades of the yogic definition of man as the universe in microcosm. Through both man and the earth is believed to run a like axis. Along man's axis—the spinal column—are strung several vibratory centres in a descending order that are key to all his functions. These Americans, echoing the Biblical account, visualize the making of man in the Creator's 'Own Image'. Then, after closing of the crown centre at the top of the head, and having suffered the 'fall', man starts his gradual ascent back upward, till he is able to eventually become 'whole' again by merging in the Source. In the ancient Chinese theory, there is the concept of *Yin* and *Yang*, which are not absolute but relative. *Yin* and *Yang* are the opposites that make the whole. *Yin* is cold, dark and female while *Yang* is hot, light and male. Neither of them can exist in isolation or without motion.

The interaction of *Yin* and *Yang* produces *Qi*—the bipolar energy. Life is possible only because of *Qi* and body, mind and emotion are all its manifestations.

In simple words, *Kundalini* is a latent bio-electric energy current that lies at the base of the spine and unknown to us, controls the output and quality of *prana* or the life force. Essentially, *Kundalini* is a vivifying and transforming process that heals psychologically and physiologically, galvanizes the neurological pathways and accesses hitherto unknown channels of the brain and nervous system. Increased creativity, heightened awareness, greater inner poise and energized spirit are all manifestations of the active *Kundalini* phenomenon. In the yoga theory within every human being, there lies this divine *Kundalini-shakti*. This energy has an external as well as an internal aspect. The external aspect sustains our worldly life, while the internal aspect brings us glimpses of the higher truths. *Kundalini* is *Shakti* or the Supreme energy, worshipped by the *Siddhas* as the Mother of the Universe. In the form of *Shakti,* She is the consort of *Shiva*—the Male Principle—and as such, the dynamic aspect of the formless Absolute. She is the substratum of our lives too; with Her external flow, She activates our mind and the senses and thus controls all our activities. It is the *Kundalini* Who senses through our ears, eyes and the tongue. It is She who supports the breath and the heart beat. However, it is the inner aspect of the working of the *Kundalini* that needs to be our focus. The inner *Kundalini*, normally lies dormant, thus concealing Her true nature from us. Her true nature, once revealed through yoga–practices, illumines the mind, the intellect and also Herself. Scriptures aver that no matter how many times the mantra is repeated, no matter how much penances are performed, and no matter how much yoga practised, Self realization is not possible as long as the inner *Kundalini* is dormant. Beneath the yoga philosophy lies practical advice as to how the *Kundalini* energy can be awakened by a systematic practice of yogic techniques, including *Asanas*,

Pranayamas, Mudras, Bandhas and the *Mantra.* The safest and easiest method, however, is said to be through *Shaktipat,* or the descent of the spiritual energy from a *Siddha*, of which I would speak later.

Coming to the West, much of Walt Whitman's poetry is said to be the outpouring of and about an active *Kundalini.* C. G. Jung was also keenly interested in the *Kundalini*, and wrote a paper under the title '*The Realities of Practical Psychotherapy*', in which he sees the origin and course of psychopathological disorders in terms of the *Kundalini Chakras.* Jung went so far as to say:

> "*When you succeed in the awakening of* kundlini *so that she starts to move out of her mere potentiality, you necessarily start a world which is totally different from our world: it is a world of eternity.*"

Lilian Silburn, Director of Research at the National Scientific Research Institute in Paris, and an eminent researcher in Kashmir Shaivism, has in her book, '*Kundalini—The Energy of the Depths*', thrown much needed light on *Kundalini* in modern times. She has also rightly cautioned the reader against undertaking uneducated attempts at awakening the dormant energies, which when not properly channelled, can wreak havoc. Perhaps the most comprehensive account of the *Kundalini* however, is to be found in Gopikrishna's (1903-1984) autobiography, *Kundalini: Evolutionary Energy in Man,* which in its first English edition contained a psychological commentary by James Hillman. A native of Kashmir, Gopikrishna after years of meditation, experienced a profound awakening of the "Serpent Power" and his works did much to familiarize the West with *Kundalini-yoga.* However, modern psychology would have to do a lot of 'soul searching' before it can come anywhere near a basic understanding of the esoteric *Kundalini* processes. In this sense, modern psychology is yet to 'arrive' in the manner modern physics and new medicine have already done. Meanwhile, the yoga seeker can wait for science to give the *Kundalini* energy its due, at his own peril.

To Recap

1. Death has been widely researched in recent times, with significant evidence emerging that human consciousness survives cessation of the physical body.
2. In the yoga theory, our physical body is but the 'densest' of a series of conjoined bodies that are neatly arranged as invisible sheaths in a descending order of coarseness.
3. The subtle bodies are a complex network of *nadis* and *chakras* that are energized by *prana*, and in a heightened state, by the *Kundalini–shakti*.
4. *Nadis* are the psycho-energetic pathways that carry *prana* or the primal life force throughout the subtle body, and are said to number 720 millions in the human form.
5. The three most important *nadis* are the *ida* or the cold current, the *pingala* or the hot current, and *susumna,* the even current. Unlike the *ida* and the *pingala* that roughly correspond to the parasympathetic and the sympathetic, the susumna is generally closed in most human beings.
6. *Chakras* are the seven psycho-spiritual energy centres strung along the spinal axis or the susumna, that are the key to all our physical, mental and spiritual activity.
7. *Kundalini–shakti* is the dormant Serpent Power or the latent bio-electric energy–powerhouse wherein lie the great secrets of healing and yoga.

VI. Planets and Free Will

"To lose one parent, Mr. Worthing, may be regarded as a misfortune; to lose both looks like carelessness."

—OSCAR WILDE

It is now no big news to the New Age brigade that yoga is man's best bet against all physical and mental disabilities, going by the exponential growth of the yoga cult in these 'happening' times. And few among the new converts would outright reject the thesis that yoga is holistic, in the sense that it impacts man's body, mind and spirit simultaneously. Yet, physical diseases are only a fraction of man's colossal suffering in a lifetime. Poverty, litigation, accidents, neglect, betrayal, death of near and dear ones—tragedy confronts us in all conceivable ways, preventing us from living life 'wholly' and by definition, from enjoying 'health'. Yoga would, therefore, be far from a holistic solution to man's problems if its healing powers were confined to man's physical and mental infirmities. Should that be the case, there could hardly be any justification for inclusion of a full chapter on '*Planets and Free Will*' in a book on yoga—'the science of healing'. It would be naive nonetheless, to presume that the *law of karma* which is at the root of yoga, manifested itself only in the realm of man's physical well-being or the lack of it. Some of the most ardent votaries of yoga that I have met, including many yoga professionals, have been uneasy with its 'unscientific' claims to bringing divine succour and shield to mankind. These educated, well meaning people would readily believe stories that regular practice of yoga/meditation revived a man dying of cancer, but they would, quite understandably, scoff at claims that a sincere practice of yoga saved another gentlemen's life by enabling him to escape a potentially fatal road accident. Surely, a speeding lorry on the highway behind your back does not discriminate between a physically sturdy and a sickly man and would kill the victim in a run-over case regardless. Death, injury or reprieve would here appear to be a matter of destiny rather than of individual health, and yoga could ostensibly be of little help, save in the seemingly unlikely event of the yoga–process influencing nothing less than destiny itself. This brings us to the vexed question of pre-destination and free will. I for one, after years of doubt and introspection, am now convinced of one thing; inasmuch as it draws sustenance from sources divine, any serious and sustained practice of Yoga has divine consequences for the practitioner (*Sadhaka)* by unearthing, for him, the hitherto latent dimensions of higher life and existence. However, before we discuss this subject any further, I would first like to say a few words about astrology.

Astrology: Destiny Deciphered?

Contrary to the popular notion, astrology is much more than fortune telling just as Yoga is much more extensive than *hatha-yoga.* A good astrological analysis of an individual's life based on his birth particulars would of course contain predictions; but it would also attempt to make a detailed three-dimensional study of his personality. It also gives one enough insight into one's inherent abilities and infirmities so as to enable him to suitably amend his life-style and thus significantly *heal* his future within the four walls of his destiny.

In today's world, an overt belief in astrology is generally considered a sign of superstition and mental weakness. Yet, few can resist the temptation of having a glance at the monthly astrological predictions that are now providing succour to almost all Hindi/English periodicals in India. (Sometime back, the editor of a reputed English magazine went on record that it was the generally accepted practice among editors of most Indian magazines to casually lift one of the older issues of the same magazine and publish the corresponding month's astrological forecast all over again in the current issue, just in case the astrologer on their rolls defaulted. No wonder, K. N. Rao calls monthly/weekly astrological forecasts in periodicals the 'opium of people'!) An excessive dependence on astrology is indeed avoidable, especially in view of the surfeit of ignorant, unscrupulous 'fortune makers' all around. Planets—contrary to the general belief—only indicate the future events and do not in any way cause them. Future events are said to be the direct consequence of one's own past karmas, and the course of their unfolding can be 'traced' by tracking the movements of all nine planets put together. A student of science can easily tell the vital distinction between correlation and causation. For instance, the sun's exact location and trajectory can be arrived at by making a close scrutiny of our shadows in the sun; this however does not mean that the shadows are causing the movements of the sun itself.

Is man then a maker of his own destiny or is he eternally consigned to its thralldom? Given the vast ramifications of this issue, and the fact that they ought to be of immediate concern to any genuine yoga-practitioner, I think it would be in order to explain the views of some of the greatest minds, ancient and modern, on the subject. I would start with an astrologer of unquestionable credentials, and follow it up with thoughts of two fully illumined modern yogis, before rounding up with sage Patanjali.

K. N. Rao

An eminent astrologer and a spiritualist of high standing, K.N. Rao's pioneering research in these fields together with his remarkably high astrological 'strike rate', has earned him an international acclaim. I can count myself among the lucky few who have enjoyed some personal rapport with him over the last few years. And although by his own admission, he is now 'tired of astrology', more so of giving predictions, he has been considerate enough to respond to my queries—both astrological and spiritual—concerning me and the larger issues. (One of his most remarkable predictions concerning me was made in 1997 when he told me that my this book would be published in 2001!) In his writings, this great astrologer seems to have taken, to the layman at least, a baffling stand on this issue. At one point in his book *Yogis, Destiny and the Wheel of Time*, he indicates that *graha-shanti is a natural occurrence in the life of a sadhaka,* implying that yoga not only changes the practitioner from within but also *rearranges* the seemingly external forces of destiny that enveloped him. Citing an example, he discusses the horoscope of a serious *sadhaka* whose birth charts indicated serious afflictions, even death, but who instead got away with minor hiccups in that critical phase of his life. Yet, at another place in the same book, he clarifies that *nothing ever happens to a man, that is not contained in his birth horoscope. One could hope to modify one's fate by different means upto a point*, he seems to argue, *but it could be done only within the broad parameters laid down for him at the precise moment of his birth.* Citing an example from everyday life, this time in the context of *japa-yoga*, Rao implies that the mantra meditation could give you the inner strength to face a nasty boss at the workplace while doling out little hope that the boss could be done away with altogether. So what was in store for the *sadhaka* in this case—a mere augmentation of the inner reservoirs to deal with the same boss, or an altogether new or reformed one? "You cannot change your boss"—one never tires of hearing this cliché at the work place in times of unpleasantness. This common refrain makes eminent sense in normal life, but leaves a volley of unanswered questions in its trail, when we are dealing with the ''supernormal''.

Although Rao, busy as ever, has not been in the best of health of late, he could still spare time for me and my discerning readers enabling me to include his thoughts even as this book went to the press. He spoke with his usual candour and verve on such vexed issues as *Reiki*, *asana-siddhi*, vegetarianism and yes, destiny and free will. Rao agreed that meditation, in particular *japa-yoga,* had a most healing influence on one's future by way of *graha-shanti*, or propitiation of planets. He rather tersely, described the three-fold influence as *katana* (nullifying), *ghatana* (dilution) and *uthana* (transcendence). He went on to explain that serious meditation enables the individual to gradually overcome astrologically indicated suffering in three distinct ways. Some future troubles that are of minor nature and *likely* to happen, get annulled altogether (*katana*). A few major reversals that are more deep rooted and bound to confront us, get diluted to a point where they are relatively easier to absorb (*ghatana*). The rest of the suffering that remains undiminished and lies in wait to defiantly rear its head in future, is the underframe that silhouettes the basic structure of our life, and by all accounts, is too deep-seated to be shaken off. A true yoga-practitioner however, is able to loosen the hold of even this class of suffering by rising in God-consciousness and identifying more with the spirit than with the flesh (*uthana*). That Rao, the astrologer, is somewhat sceptical of even a theoretical possibility of Yoga changing one's destiny upside down is understandable. For, determinism and not free will, can be the genuine ideological support of astrology—any attempt to foresee/foretell the future made sense only if such a future 'already existed'. The important thing to note however, is his admission that yoga at its best was still capable of removing all conscious suffering insofar as it 'touched' you and me.

Yukteswar Giri

In his *Autobiography of a Yogi*, Paramahansa Yogananda extensively quotes his Guru, Swami Yukteswar Giri, in the chapter *Outwitting the Stars*. By all accounts, Swami Yukteswar was an authority on scriptures and more importantly, he was a Siddha. His views on the matter are, therefore, of no mean significance. While advising Yogananda to have an open and inquiring mind towards astrology, he underlines the importance of *graha-shanti* as part of Yoga, over and above the obvious importance of performing good karmas. According to him, quite aside from the *karmic* principle, there are certain mechanical aspects to the working of human destiny that brooked mechanical solutions such as wearing of gems, metallic bangles or plant roots (*jadis*) next to the skin. Undoubtedly, wearing of precious gem or a semiprecious bangle was not quite a good karma in itself and if it could influence the future events, as Yukteswar Giri says it does, then there was certainly something more to man's destiny than the *law of karma* as we understand. Yogananda in fact, gives a fascinating account of how his bout of illness that was 'destined' to continue for six months, was reduced to a mere 24 days with the aid of a metallic '*kara*' (helped, one suspects, by the Siddha Guru's own blessings that the modest Guru was apt to disown). Savour then, the essence of wisdom flowing from Yogananda's Guru:

"*It is not a question of* belief: *the scientific attitude one should take on any subject is whether it is* true. *The law of gravitation worked as efficiently before Newton as after him. The cosmos would be fairly chaotic if its laws could not operate without the sanction of human belief.*

"Charlatans have brought the ancient stellar science to its present disrepute. Astrology is too vast, both mathematically and philosophically, to be rightly grasped except by men of profound understanding. If ignoramuses misread the heavens, and see there a scrawl instead of a script, that is to be expected in this imperfect world. One should not dismiss the wisdom with the 'wise'.

"All parts of creation are linked together and interchange their influences. The balanced rhythm of the universe is rooted in

reciprocity".... "Man, in his human aspect, has to combat two sets of forces – first, the tumults within his being, caused by the admixture of earth, water, fire, air, and ethereal elements; second, the outer disintegrating powers of nature. So long as man struggles with his mortality, he is affected by the myriad mutations of heaven and earth.

"Astrology is the study of man's response to planetary stimuli. The stars have no conscious benevolence or animosity; they merely send forth positive and negative radiations. Of themselves, these do not help or harm humanity, but offer a lawful channel for the outward operation of cause-effect equilibriums that each man has set into motion in the past.

"A child is born on that day and that hour when the celestial rays are in mathematical harmony with his individual karma. His horoscope is a challenging portrait, revealing his unalterable past and its probable future results. But the natal chart can be rightly interpreted only by men of intuitive wisdom: these are few.

" The message boldly blazoned across the heavens at the moment of birth is not meant to emphasize fate – the result of past good and evil – but to arouse man's will to escape from his universal thralldom. What he has done, he can undo. None other than himself was the instigator of the causes of whatever effects are now prevalent in his life. He can overcome any limitation, because he created it by his own actions in the first place, and because he possesses spiritual resources that are not subject to planetary pressure.

"Superstitious awe of astrology makes one an automation, slavishly dependent on mechanical guidance. The wise man defeats his planets – which is to say, his past – by transferring his allegiance from the creation to the Creator. The more he realizes his unity with Spirit, the less he can be dominated by matter. The soul is ever free; it is deathless because birthless. It cannot be regimented by stars.

"Man is *a soul, and* has *a body. When he properly places his sense of identity, he leaves behind all compulsive patterns. So long as he remains confused in his ordinary state of spiritual*

amnesia, he will know the subtle fetters of environmental law. "God is Harmony; the devotee who attunes himself will never perform any action amiss. His activities will be correctly and naturally timed to accord with astrological law. After deep prayer and meditation he is in touch with his divine consciousness; there is no greater power than inward protection".

".......By a number of means – by prayer, by will power, by yoga meditation, by consultation with saints, by use of astrological bangles – the adverse effect of past wrongs can be minimized or nullified".

Yogananda concludes by adding his own incisive observation–

> *"The deeper the Self – realization of a man, the more he influences the whole Universe by his subtle spiritual vibrations, and the less he himself is affected by the phenomenal flux".*

(Paramahansa Yogananda, *Autobiography of a Yogi*. Los Angeles: Self-Realization Fellowship, 1998)

A less picturesque, yet equally illuminating account of predestination and free will comes from Swami Muktananda, another great Siddha and authority on scriptures, not unfamiliar to the West. Personally, the Muktananda approach to *Sadhana* and operation of free will has been the most enduring influence in my life ever since I took to yoga, and with each passing year I am left with a lighter and lighter baggage of doubt notwithstanding the trials and tribulations of day–to-day existence. Briefly, the Muktananda thesis which essentially is the Siddha Yoga approach, is as under.

Muktananda

In astrology, there are all together twelve houses in an individual's horoscope that represent the sum total of his life, or rather his 'lives' given the fact that he was born many times before and was likely (though by no means certain) to be born many times again. Each of these twelve houses represents many aspects of his life, but is most representative of one key area. The representation is something like this–

(i)	Ist house	—	Self, Health, Longevity
(ii)	2nd	—	Wealth
(iii)	3rd	—	Valour, Coborns
(iv)	4th	—	Lands, Conveyances, Mother
(v)	5th	—	Progeny, Worship
(vi)	6th	—	Disease, Debt, Enemies
(vii)	7th	—	Spouse
(viii)	8th	—	Death
(ix)	9th	—	Fortune
(x)	10th	—	Profession, Income
(xi)	11th	—	Gains
(xii)	12th	—	Losses, *Moksha*

Quite emphatically, Swami Muktananda declares that *Shaktipat* meditation, which is the most natural and concentrated form of yoga, has the greatest conceivable corrective and curative influence on the practitioner's whole destiny as symbolized by the twelve houses. As such this Yoga is theoretically capable of enabling the *sadhaka* to completely transcend the limitations imposed upon him by his moment of physical birth. Significantly, *diksha* as the entrance-way to *Shaktipat* meditation is said to be the *second birth* of the subject making him a *dvija* or the *twice born.* As one goes deeper and deeper in this esoteric meditation, the twelve houses are getting purified one by one, starting from the first house. Accordingly, areas of weakness and negativity in the subject's destiny as indicated by planetary afflictions become muted or removed altogether in that order. Thus, at the beginning of the *Sadhana*, the practitioner is blessed with excellent health and greater life force. As the yogic influence moves to the second house, the *sadhaka* becomes rich and capable of charity. With the purification of the third house, the *sadhaka* becomes firm in the face of life's challenges. In this way, the reformative process of the superimposition of the Divine Will on mundane existence goes on till *Sadhana* permeates the twelfth house, at which stage the *sadhaka* becomes liberated, having exhausted all karmas. Briefly, the revelations of Paramahansa Muktananda on the intricate interplay of destiny and free will, as viewed from the prism of astrology, can be summed up as below:

(a) *Astrology traces the impact of the zodiac's twelve signs on one's life, assessing the relative positions of the planets in these signs and signifying thus one's good or bad fortune.*

(b) *It is a science rooted in scriptures that essentially shows how our karmas of past births determine our present and future in the current life in the form of destiny* (prarabdha).

(c) *Those who have a weak* dhana sthana *(house of wealth) live a life of wants, and those who have an afflicted* putra sthana *(house of offspring) get wayward children, or none at all.*

(d) *Likewise, those who don't have a pure* jaya sthana *(house of conjugal association) do not get happiness through matrimony. And so on and so forth, till the last of the twelve houses is reached.*

(e) *Yet, a* sadhaka *who does the mantra meditation with love and conviction, gradually comes to derive the maximum benefits of all houses overcoming planetary afflictions.*

(f) *As* sadhana, *one by one purifies all houses, the* sadhaka *comes to be blessed with good health* (tanu sthana), *prosperity* (dhana sthana), *valour* (parakrama sthana), *erudition* (vidya sthana) *and so on till mantra meditation penetrates the twelfth and final house signifying liberation* (moksha).

(g) *Mantra meditation is therefore a veritable wish fulfilling tree* (kalpa vriksha)—*a gem that brings all things desired* (parama chintamani).

The Roots

Summing up, we must go back to Patanjali and see what he has to say on human suffering and deliverance. The sage identifies five hindrances or *kleshas*: nescience (*avidya*), 'I-am-ness' (*asmita*), attachment (*raga*), aversion (*dvesha*) and the will-to-live (*abhinivesha*). The *Yoga Sutra* recognises these *kleshas* as the breeding ground of the subliminal activators (*samskaras*) that form the "karmic deposit" (*karmashaya*). The *karmashaya*, in turn, determines the span and quality of man's present and future lives. And the manifest purpose of Patanjali Yoga is to achieve a gradual attenuation or 'thinning out' (*tanu-karana*) of the *kleshas* until these are completely obliterated in realization. From an astrological point of view, one's natal chart symbolises the *karmashaya*. And it is the process of thinning out of the *kleshas* as a result of yoga-practice, that is reflected in the purging of zodiacal houses. Patanjali's revelations on the riddle of determinism vs. free will can then, be summed up as below:

(i) *Nescience* (avidya), *'I am'ness* (asmita), *passion* (raga), *aversion* (vidvesha) *and the will-to-live* (abhinivesha) *are the five hindrances.*

(ii) *The latent deposit of karma has its root in the hindrances and may be felt in a birth seen or unseen.*

(iii) *So long as the root exists, there will be a three-fold fruition: birth, length-of-life and kind-of-experience.*

(iv) *Self-castigation, study and devotion to God* (Ishwara) *are the Yoga of action.*

(v) *When the hindrances are sufficiently attenuated through Yoga of action and finally cut off, the latent deposits begin to dry up.*

(vi) *Although the latent-deposits are endless and their period of ripening unsettled, they cannot bear fruit when they are burned in seed form by Elevation* (prasamkhyana).

While theoretically, every yoga practitioner can purify all the twelve houses in succession and thus transcend all finitude, the ground reality is that this accomplishment is largely the prerogative of a Siddha. For most men liberation, going by the scriptural wisdom, is many life times away. In ordinary living, yoga can nonetheless, be said to have served its purpose of *healing the future* reasonably well, if in this life, we ensure for ourselves physical well-being, enough longevity, a degree of material cushioning, purposeful living and happiness through children and conjugal life. It is also worth mentioning here that the yoga process influencing the twelve houses in succession does not quite mean that at any given time it influences one house to the exclusion of eleven others. As a matter of fact, like everything else in the universe, the curative influence is holistic, i.e., it is impacting all the twelve houses all the time in varying degrees with their being no room for any rigid compartmentalization.

To Recap

1. Physical diseases are a tiny fraction of man's suffering in a life time that is rooted in the retributive law of karma.
2. Yoga, in order to be a holistic remedy, must go well beyond physical well being and be able to rearrange karmic grooves themselves.
3. Astrology is the study of man's response to positive and negative planetary stimuli, which in themselves have no conscious benevolence or animosity.
4. A sustained practice of Yoga enables man to access his Free Will and thereby triumph over many negative aspects of his destiny as signified by planets.
5. An advanced yoga practitioner, specially one blessed with *Shaktipat* initiation, can truly defeat his stars through the soul force, and fulfil himself in all conceivable ways.

VII. Shaktipat: The 'Lightning' Yoga

"Consider the lilies of the field, how they grow; they toil not, neither do they spin."

—MATTHEW, 6:28

Throughout the book, I have been cautioning the reader not to look for shortcuts and instant hits in Yoga. Now that the point is hopefully driven home, let me have the pleasure of contradicting myself by introducing you to a kind of Yoga that can give you a real shortcut. While all other types of yoga practices need you to be toiling, persevering and relentlessly on your toes all the time, this yoga is literally 'lightning quick'. It is capable of changing you in a flash even if the outer manifestations of the profound change brought about thus, take time to emerge. In this most complete of all yoga practices, you have to neither struggle with yourself, nor seek anyone's regular assistance. For, this Yoga, once started, rapidly unfolds on its own and begins to heal you almost *in spite of yourself*. The metaphor of lightning is not very far-fetched, since this method makes use of transmission of a Siddha's lightning-like energy or *Shakti* to 'electrocute' you through his touch, glance, thought or word. Since this yoga begins with *Shaktipat* (descent of energy) and quickly ushers in the meditative state, I will simply call this *Shaktipat–yoga*.

It is often said that true meditation is never done, it *happens*. Likewise, the great secret of yoga lies in its complete effortlessness and spontaneity; you do not start yoga, but yoga gets you started. So long as you are pushing and prodding yourself into various yogic practices—*asana*, *pranayama* etc.—you are only probing the fringes. The key to success in yoga lies in painstakingly piercing the rind that protects the 'nut', and getting 'one full bite'. After that, there is no looking back; things start falling in place on their own and in a chain reaction, you find yourself practising yoga with ever-increasing vigour without much trying. The nuclear physicists describe the most crucial stage in the nuclear power-generating process as 'going critical'. *Criticality* is something that once triggered, sets off a controlled chain reaction that is self-sustaining. In the New Age science, when the boundaries of nuclear physics and yoga theory are merging, one could say that in yoga also, the all important thing for the practitioner to patiently wait for, is for the yoga process 'to go critical', after which he has to just cooperate with the cosmic forces that are unleashed from within:

> "We do not know how it happens, but *Sadhana* follows the seeker and *Samadhi* itself goes in search of his mind."
>
> —*Jnaneshwar Maharaj*

I would illustrate this with an example. Think of a tribal who has somehow strayed onto a forlorn city highway and stumbles against an unknown object that in fact is a Mercedes—keys dangling, doors open and no one else around. The weary tribal wants to get back to the safety of the woods fast, but knows that the familiar forests are an arduous 40 km-walk up the highway. He looks longingly at the four-wheeled wonder—"if only one could carry this beauty to the jungles"! He awes at the sleek body, admires it from a distance, and then pushes it with all his might, only to realize that it just won't move. In disgust, he leaves the damned thing behind and resumes his dreary walk that, given the odds, may or may not restore him to his habitat. In a couple of hours, there comes another tribal with the same predicament. He too bumps against the Mercedes with the same longing thought—"if only one could return to safety by managing the 40 km. highway walk with this beautiful thing in tow"! Only this chap turns out to be luckier—he spots a neatly dressed stranger around, who in fact is none other than the driver of the car. The intelligent man quickly understands the plight of the waylaid tribal, as also his fascination for the car. In a benevolent and playful gesture, he hands over the keys to the tribal, puts him behind the driving wheel, gets him to switch on the engine and make a move. There is no holding back thereafter; the wonder-struck tribal enjoys himself to the hilt with the clutch, accelerator, the wheel and the brake, on the open highway—all under the watchful eyes of the driver. Sitting cozily in the bucket seat, and 'doing nothing', he yet covers the 40 km. stretch in a jiffy and reaches his destination. As he takes leave of his saviour, he has had no bruises, no fatigue, no encounters with snakes and tigers. What lingers on is a sense of gratitude for the 'master', the relief of home coming and a boundless joy of having tamed the big, beautiful machine.

Before I go on, I would like my reader to appreciate this. If we put ourselves in place of the tribal, then the tribal is us, the Mercedes is our human form, the driver is the Guru and the ignition switch is *Shaktipat*. When Jnaneshwar Maharaj talks of '*Sadhana following the seeker*' and '*Samadhi going in search of his mind*', he is essentially talking of the chauffeur–guided Mercedes carrying the tribal all the way to his goal in an enjoyable ride. Contrast this with the uninspiring and ungainly sight of the tribal pushing the dead weight of the Mercedes all the way back home. Now, in order that we understand *Shaktipat* we have to recollect from the previous chapters, that yoga is all about a part–systematic, part-spontaneous process of awakening of the latent inner energies that reside in the *Kundalini*.

Shaktipat

True yoga, therefore, starts only when the *Kundalini-shakti* is awakened. This *Shakti* can be awakened in a number of ways—through intense *bhakti* or devotion to God, through rigorous *hatha-yoga* exercises, or through chanting and *pranayama.* Very occasionally, a ripe seeker can also experience a spontaneous awakening thanks to his spiritual 'opening balance' in the shape of yogic practices performed in past lives. Scriptures describe the different ways in which *Shakti* can be awakened. The sweetest and safest method of awakening the *Shakti* however, is through *Shaktipat* (literally, 'the descent of spiritual energy') from a Siddha Guru. Simply put, *Shaktipat* is the rather mysterious process whereby a deserving disciple receives a Siddha Guru's fully awakened spiritual charge or *Shakti*, thus sparking off the disciple's own hitherto locked-up *Kundalini*. Seers down the ages have been privy to this sacred, unbroken tradition of *Shaktipat* that runs back in time to the birth of humanity itself. From time immemorial, it has been passed on from one Siddha Guru to his disciple, then by the disciple–turned Guru to his own disciple, and so on till this day. Nor is *Shaktipat* an exclusive preserve of the Hindu tradition. The Old and the New Testaments, for example, are replete with instances of Jesus laying his hands over someone and suffusing him with a surge of bliss and love with a single transforming touch. The New Testament gives the blind man's account of his miracle-healing, "I once was blind, but now I see." In the Oriental tradition, the most well-known instances of spiritual transmutation through *Shaktipat* are those of Swami Vivekananda (by Ramakrishna Paramahansa), Kabir (from an accidental touch of Swami Ramananda's feet), and Jalaluddin Rumi, the Persian mystic-poet (by Shams-i–Tabriz, the maverick medieval saint).

The *Shakti* resides in the Guru's flesh and blood in such abundance and fury that it is being continuously exuded in the atmosphere around him, and is getting absorbed by articles of his daily use. Amir Khusrau, the Persian poet–philosopher is said to have instantly become restored to the Self from touching the shoes of the great Sufi saint, Hazrat

Nizammudin. K. N. Rao recounts how his Guru, Swami Parmananda Saraswati, during his last days, lovingly gave him a fruit to eat—one that was 'charged' with the Guru's *Shakti*. It is another matter that Rao selflessly gave it in turn to his mother who was a great astrologer to start with, and who became completely clairvoyant upon eating the charged fruit. K. N. Rao also writes of his *Shaktipat* experiences with another great Siddha, Nagaridas Baba, sitting next to whom at Vrindavana was literally such a 'mind-blowing' experience that K. N. Rao was never able to properly converse with him for any length of time.

In the literature on Swami Muktananda, there comes a hilarious, yet poignant account of how a veterinary doctor, while examining Muktananda's ailing lapdog, got 'electrocuted' by the *Shakti* that had gathered in the animal through the constant hugging of Swami Muktananda. The poor doctor did not know what had hit him. (When Muktananda later came to know of the victim's plight, he jokingly remarked that the doctor had now become an initiated disciple of the lapdog! Siddhas, as it transpires, are not lacking in sense of humour.) In yet another interesting instance, Swami Satyananda, founder of the world famous Bihar School of Yoga at Munger, narrates how, while approaching Paramahansa Nityananda (Muktananda's Guru), he received 'electric shocks' and felt like touching a live cable as he ventured closer. In case of my own Guru (Hans Baba), Amrita Pritam, the noted Indian poetess has written how her chronic and seemingly incurable problem of arthritis vanished in the presence of the great Siddha who did no more than tap his *Machan*; more of that later.

Ripe seekers like K. N. Rao and Swami Satyananda receive '*darshana*' and blessings of several *Siddhas* in their life time, and can, therefore, recount a great many instances of *Shaktipat* experiences from their tryst with a great many *Siddhas*. My own *Shaktipat* experiences spring from my exposure to one single Siddha, Hans Baba and my briefly describing them in this book is intended to motivate many a reader to follow suit. The significance of such *Shaktipat*-encounters from the recipient's point of view, can be gauged from the scriptural saying that *it takes the accumulated* 'punyas' *(good karmas) of countless births for one to be blessed even once with the* 'darshana' *of a Siddha.* Underlying this is the belief that even a 'chance' meeting—let alone *Shaktipat* initiation—with a Siddha is potentially a turning point in a man's life, washing away as it does, a considerable chunk of one's accumulated bad karmas (*papa*). Indeed, one of the most effective astrological measures of '*graha-shanti*' is said to come in the form of *darshana* and blessings of a Siddha, whose powers to triumph over his own destiny as well as that of his supplicants, has never been doubted in the Indian tradition.

Initiation

Shakti can descend from the *Siddha* Guru to the seeker, in the process of *diksha* or spiritual initiation in one of four ways—by touch (*Sparsha diksha*), by word (*Mantra diksha*), by Guru's look (*Drik diksha*) and by Guru's thought (*Manas diksha*). The *Siddha* Guru is a virtual powerhouse of spiritual energy; his physical body is crackling with so much *Kundalini* energy that the disciple gets *Shaktipat* initiation by a mere touch. The Guru may touch the seeker's body at one or all of three main places—at the space between the two eyebrows or the third eye centre (*ajna chakra*), near the heart centre (the *anahata chakra*) and near the *muladhara* or the base of the spine. The *Siddha* Guru's utterances have the supreme divine power (*Paravani*) and therefore his whispering of the 'word' or *mantra* into the ears of the disciple results in mantra–initiation. The Guru has repeated the mantra long enough during his *Sadhana* to have cracked the power of the mantra and is able to charge it with a living force. The gaze of a Guru is invariably fixed inward on the Self, notwithstanding the external appearance that may suggest otherwise (*shambhavi mudra*). His look therefore, radiates the power of Consciousness which when absorbed by the disciple, can result in *Drik diksha*. To the ripe seeker however, *Shaktipat* initiation can come even in the form of a thought, or *Manas diksha*.

When experience of the Self comes to the disciple in a flash, through the Guru's touch, word, look or thought, this is called *Shambhavi diksha*. The initiation of Kabir and Vivekananda falls in this category. This, however, is the rarest type of *Shaktipat* meant for seekers of the highest order. For the less endowed, scriptures speak of all together twenty seven categories of *Shaktipat* in a descending order of intensity. The *Shakti* is nonetheless identical—it is only the people who defer in their capacity to hold it. Each person, therefore, gets *Shaktipat* initiation in strict accordance with his temperament and past karmas.

Effects of Initiation

Shaktipat is the quintessential yoga because it contains all other yogas in their most concentrated form. Scriptures say that all the penances performed, all the *mantras* recited and all the yoga practised are not enough to let us realize the Self as long as the *Kundalini* energy is not let loose. *Hatha-yoga*, *Raja-yoga*, *Bhakti-yoga*, *Mantra-yoga*, *Laya-yoga* and yoga of all other hues occur spontaneously once the *Kundalini* energy gets activated through *Shaktipat*. All the seeker is required to do thereafter is to cooperate with the unfolding *Shakti*. By not neglecting *Sadhana* and through meditation, love for the Guru and a reasonably disciplined life, the practitioner can increase the *Shakti* manifold. In this, the seeker does not have to overly stretch himself since post initiation, love for God and the orientation for yogic practices arise in him on their own.

Readers would recall that of the 720 million '*nadis*' that are believed to constitute the human body, the three most important are said to be the '*ida*'(the cold or 'moon' channel), '*pingala*' (the hot or 'solar' channel) and the '*susumna*' (the central channel). *Ida* and *pingala* are active in every human body, as the breath comes in and goes out through these two *nadis*. The most important *nadi,* however—the *susumna*—lies dormant in most of us. It is located between the *ida* and *pingala* and runs along the spinal column. The *susumna,* unknown to us, controls all life's activities and all other *nadis*. It originates near the *muladhara*—seat of the dormant *Kundalini* coiled up in three-and–a-half folds—and extends right up to the *sahasrara*—the crown centre in the head that is supposedly the abode of the supreme Shiva.

The karmas of past lives are said to be stored in the *susumna*, which in turn trigger the various states—lust, envy, anger, inspiration etc. Peace, knowledge, compassion and like other yogic qualities are believed to reside in the higher realms of the *susumna*. The lower *susumna* stores such unyogic states as fear, insecurity and anger. Once the *Shakti* is awakened, all the past karmas come to the fore. As they surface, we experience them. As such, it is quite possible that just after receiving *Shaktipat*, one feels very low or negative. It is however, a sure sign that the awakened *Shakti* is ejecting all the karmas of past births. Occasionally, one may even start crying incessantly for no apparent reason in a 'cathartic release'.

When the *Kundalini* first becomes active as a result of *Shaktipat,* one may literally become sluggish and sleepy. However, as *Kundalini* travels up the *susumna*, the body is rapidly purged of all impurities and completely transformed in order that it can hold the full impact of the unfolding *Shakti*. Ayurveda attributes all physiological disorders to the imbalances in the three bodily humours ('*tridoshas*')—*Vata* (wind), *Pitta* (bile) and *Kapha* (phlegm). The active *Kundalini* inspires the various yogic '*kriyas*' to purify all 720 million *nadis* of these imbalances and rejuvenate them with more abundant flow of *prana*.

Latent germs of diseases may come out leading to a

temporary suffering of the disease that nonetheless, is the sign of an imminent, permanent cure. Involuntary shaking and swaying of the limbs and the torso, frenetic spinning of the head, and such other *kriyas* may be experienced on their own. Likewise, one may find oneself automatically performing different *hatha-yogic asanas*, *mudras*, *bandhas* and *pranayamas*. All these are the powerful purificatory influence of the active *Kundalini* that is an unalloyed blessing for the seeker's psyche and physique. Blocks are then removed, traumas repaired and addictions cast aside as life becomes much more meaningful and vibrant.

When the *hatha-yogic asanas* are practised consciously with the aid of our limited knowledge of the physiological processes involved, one is never quite certain as to exactly which *asanas*, *mudras*, *bandhas* and *pranayamas* are needed for us. For instance, *sirshasana* may be excellent for person X, but actually harmful for person Y—and yet there is no fail-safe method of determining it for sure. The greatness of the *Shaktipat*-engineered *hatha-yogic kriyas* lies in the fact that the seeker gets to practise exactly those *kriyas*—and none else—that are beneficial for his constitution.

Just like the spontaneously occurring *hatha-yogic kriyas*, other yogas also start happening spontaneously. The non-attachment of *karma-yoga*, the ecstatic devotion of *bhakti-yoga*, the higher understanding of *jnana-yoga*, the bursting out of Sanskrit hymns of *mantra-yoga* and the inner sounds and visions of *laya-yoga*—all or some of these may come about effortlessly. In the process, the *prana* (outgoing breath) and *apana* (incoming breath) become uniform and neutralized, and the breath begins to be retained inside (*Kumbhaka*). When the *prana* becomes still, the mind becomes tranquil and one fleetingly experiences the supreme bliss that is normally associated with the state of *savikalpa samadhi.*

Initiation and Worldly Life

Fears are often expressed that spiritual advancement of any

manner can come but at the expense of worldly happiness. To the unaccustomed, the very mention of the word '*diksha*' rings of *Sanyasa* or like other connotations, since reconciliation of worldly pursuits with the spiritual ideal of renunciation appears prima-facie impossible. However, it may be recalled from the earlier deliberations, that in the holistic process of yoga, the spiritual, the mental and the physical are the three interactive dimensions that blend seamlessly to form one integrated whole that outgrows all initial contradiction. The scriptures say—'*where there is realization, there are no worldly enjoyments, and where there are worldly enjoyments, there is no realization; but when one receives the grace of divinly caring Kundalini, worldly enjoyment and realization go together*'. The *rishis* or ancient seers were mostly householders who fulfilled all worldly obligations and yet became established in God–Consciousness.

As a result of *Shaktipat,* the active *Shakti* changes us for the better at every strata of our existence, and this necessarily includes our worldly life. Frustration together with a sense of futility that often overcomes us in our daily life, and gives rise to a vicious circle of failures, makes way for an attitude of optimism and daring that is more conducive to worldly success and fulfillment. The awakened *Shakti* improves our family ties and strengthens us wherever we are lacking. It also improves the memory, concentration and creativity thus making a physician, a better physician, an administrator, a better administrator and a businessman, a better businessman. To the needy, the *Kundalini-shakti* may manifest as *Lakshmi*—the Goddess of Wealth—and to others, the blessing may take the form of enhanced status and dignity. In the preceding chapter, the reader has seen how *Shaktipat–yoga,* which is the most complete and concentrated form of yoga-practice, is capable of purifying all twelve houses of the *sadhaka's* birth horoscope, and bringing him all the worldly enjoyment that was otherwise impossible. The important thing to note however, is that the worldly success brought about by yoga is not likely to be of a predatory kind, but is bound to be conducive to the welfare of those around.

The Mantra

Mantra Initiation

The *Kundalini-shakti* is an all-knowing force and post *Shaktipat*, it works within our system in the safest and the best possible manner. The great secret of *Shaktipat-yoga* is that this is never contrived or imposed. As we continue the practices, the *Shakti* flowers in the most natural way and sets us on the desired path. However, the inner *Shakti*, once it has been brought alive by the Guru, needs to be continuously nursed and whetted by the practitioner through regular meditation, a disciplined diet and moderate habits. For this reason, of the four modes of initiation, *mantra-diksha* holds the greatest promise for us. As explained, the ripest of seekers—a potential *Siddha*—gets realization of the Self in a flash as he receives the *Shakti*. A Kabir or a Vivekananda is a ready example. Next in order are the handful of very advanced seekers who get initiated in one of the four ways, and are so dedicated and motivated that the Guru's Grace brings them close to the yoga state in quick time. K. N. Rao fondly remembers how, for six months running, just after his *Shaktipat* initiation by Swami Parmananda Saraswati, he continued having clairvoyant visions of the still-to-be Indo-China war of 1962 and the bloodied aftermath!

The vast majority of the seekers however comprises yoga enthusiasts who are, quite understandably, torn between the opposites of doubt and conviction, fear and optimism, neglect and perseverance. For them to get going the chain reaction of yoga on the strength of a single *Shaktipat* experience is highly unlikely. *Shaktipat* initiation through the Guru's touch, glance or thought, however potent, is more likely to be a one-time-affair in the life of the multitude of seekers, soon to wear off and be forgotten in the din and bustle of everyday life. This category of seekers needs a more enduring form of yogic influence that comes in the form of Guru's Grace, and yet is independent of the Guru's physical presence. This vital gap is what is readily filled by the Guru's live mantra.

Mantra as Sound

"In the beginning was the Word, the Word was God and the Word was with God"—says the Bible, *"and the word was made flesh and dwelt among us....full of grace and truth."*

The *Upanishads* also state that *in the beginning, there was sound which reverberated as 'Aum', and from Aum came all existence.* In the *Bhagavad Gita,* Lord Krishna says *"Among the rituals, I am the ritual of mantra repetition."* Quantum physicist are now beginning to discover, much as the ancient seers intuitively perceived, that there is an incessant vibration that underlies all phenomena and that is the substratum of all things 'material'.

Sound has enormous power. During the school days, all of us have in our physics classes, been taught why a parading army platoon is asked to disperse while crossing a bridge, lest the powerful sound vibrations thus generated smash the bridge itself. It has also been demonstrated that a violin note with its pitch raised high enough, can shatter glass. Egyptologists have tried to unravel the mystery of the 'humanly impossible' building of pyramids by surmising that the ancient Egyptians probably sculpted and moved the gigantic stones with the aid of precisely orchestrated sound vibrations.

A mantra is Spirit captured in Sound. Each mantra comprises a combination of sounds coming from the Sanskrit alphabet that has a total of fifty letters. Arguably the most ancient of all languages, Sanskrit is believed to be 'the language of the gods'. In the New Age, it has been admitted to be structurally the most scientific and pliant of all languages for computer applications. The extremely scientific nature of the language and the script is underlined by the fact that each of the fifty alphabets and all of their combinations in the form of words, are pronounced invariably and exactly the way they are written. The Sanskrit language is therefore, seen to wed sound and form in a way no other language does. "*Since the revival of classical learning*", states the Encyclopedia Americana, "*there has been no other event in the history of culture as important as the discovery of Sanskrit (by the West) in the latter part of the 18th century.*" The Sanskrit knowing *rishis* recognized the infinite power contained in sound and in the form of *mantras,* they utilized combinations of sounds to produce particular vibrations.

Mantra as Thought

Mantras are essentially the sound-body of God. There are seed *(bija) mantras* of *Tantric* origin that have no meaning. They draw their power exclusively from their precise phonetic effect that has powerful bearing on the *Kundalini* energy through the *nadis* and the *chakras*. These *bija mantras* in chaste Sanskrit, must be pronounced with absolute precision to bear fruition—not an easy thing to accomplish for most Anglicized Indians, let alone the Westerner. More relevant and useful in our context are the *Vedic* deity mantras that have definite meaning and visual impact and that therefore, can be said to be as much of thought–configurations as distinct sound patterns. A Krishna mantra evokes powerful imagery of God with attributes, Who is loving, indwelling and mischievous. A Rama mantra on other hand, evokes image of God as a strict disciplinarian, a dignified family man with the same underlying attributes of benevolence, omniscience and omnipotence.

Unlike the *bija mantra*, the deity mantras are not double-edged in that they will either do good, or at least do no harm depending on the correctness of pronunciation. The deity mantra is capable of completely transforming us from within. Our mind, our body and everything about our existence is in fact the dense and solidified form of thought vibration.

Our external appearance of fixed identities, as modern science shows us, is an illusion. Actually, we are an ever changing 'mass' of oscillations, or an ever mutating flux of Consciousness. Whatever emotion or thought arises in the mind, therefore, impacts the mind and the body instantaneously. While doctors now readily recognize the powerful psychosomatic hold of thought over the flesh, the yoga theory views the mystifying process in its own inimitable way—thoughts descending from the mind to the *prana*, from the *prana* mingling into the blood stream, and distributing themselves via the blood stream to the entire body. Mantra—the God name—therefore, causes tremors in our inner existence, cleansing the blood, fortifying the *prana* and ridding the mind of subterranean negativity.

The 'Conscious' Mantra

Scriptures speak of there being 70 million *mantras* obtainable from different sources. However, the *mantra* in order to be really efficacious, must be a live or 'conscious' mantra. *Mantras* broadly fall in two categories—the *jada* (inert) and the *chaitanya* (conscious). A mantra received from a teacher who is not a *Siddha* or one learnt from a book is an inert mantra. This mantra has little inherent power; it is a mechanical and largely inefficacious collection of letters. A live mantra on the other hand is directly received from a *Siddha* Guru who has himself received it from his own Guru, and so on in the thriving, sacred Guru–Disciple tradition. This mantra is like red hot iron in that it carries the all-consuming fire of the Guru's realization. When whispered by the Guru into the seeker's ears, it results in immediate *Shaktipat* initiation. As the seeker–turned disciple repeats the mantra with love and devotion, first sitting next to the Guru and subsequently away from him on his own, his latent inner *Shakti* is gradually awakened ushering in the spontaneous yoga. The conscious mantra should under no circumstances be shared with any one, not even the spouse.

Mantra in Action

Just as ice, water and steam are all essentially one, in the yoga theory, thought, form and sound are the different modes of the same vibrational energy. The thought–sound continuum, with sound and thought forming the two extremes, comprises four fundamental states. Mantra repetition takes the seeker from the grossest of these states to the subtlest. As the mantra is repeated, it passes from the lower to the higher states, until it finds its way back to its source—the pure Consciousness. Speech—the sound-thought entity—is said by the scriptures to manifest, starting from the grossest, as *Vaikhari, Madhyama, Pasyanti* and *Para. Vaikhari* is the fully developed and differentiated speech that people normally engage in. This gross speech arises from a subtler level, the *Madhyama,* that originates in the throat. At the *Madhyama* stage, words are fully formed, although they have not been uttered yet. *Pasyanti,* the third stage, is the unarticulated, not fully differentiated sound that is experienced in the heart region. The origin of sound, however, lies at *Para*—the deepest, transcendental state—that is pure, unmanifest sound with no differentiation, no name, no form, no wave length. This *Paravani* is experienced in the navel centre and is the subtlest vibration from which the whole universe has emerged.

After *Shaktipat* the mantra repetition initially takes place at its densest, going on silently at the level of the tongue in *Vaikhari.* After the mantra has been thus repeated long enough, it reaches the *Madhyama* stage with subtle repetition in the throat. The mantra repetition in the throat region is said to be a thousand times more effective than repetition with the physical tongue. As the repetition is continued with faith and devotion, the mantra gradually goes deeper to the *Pasyanti* level in the heart region. One repetition at the *Pasyanti* level is equal to thousands of repetitions in the throat region. The *Pasyanti* repetition sends wave after wave of bliss up the spinal column that is roughly the path of the rising *susumna*. Eventually, the mantra with continued repetition, penetrates to the fourth and final level of *Paravani* in the navel region when its power is fully unfolded. As the mantra repetition gradually descends from the tongue level down to its source, it starts giving us unusual experiences and paranormal powers(*Siddhis*) that reach their pinnacle at the *Para* level. One who has realized the full power of the mantra, gets restored to the Self and becomes a *Siddha*. Any word uttered by the *Siddha* is therefore, *Paravani*. It is for this reason that all *Siddhas* are said to have *Vak-siddhi*, i.e., whatever they utter has the potency of a mantra and is bound to fructify.

Guru

In the beginning, I have described how in the Vedas, just as in modern science, each term is uniquely and exactly defined, being incapable of loose interpretations. The common English translation of Guru as 'teacher', in the *Vedic* context, is a misnomer since the Guru, quite unlike an instructor or a preceptor, is not the purveyor of theoretical knowledge, but the 'giver of light'. The syllable '*gu*', in Sanskrit means darkness, and the guru is *one who dispels darkness*. According to the Shaivite texts, the Supreme Reality has five cosmic functions to dispense: creation, maintenance, dissolution, concealment of the true nature of the universe and the bestowal of Grace. It is the bestowal of Grace that enables human beings to outgrow the ego–identity and realize the Self. Shaivism describes Guru as the embodiment of God's fifth cosmic function. The Guru is accordingly, the medium for this fifth cosmic process. Whether they indulge in overt teaching or not, there can be little doubt that all Gurus are teachers of the highest order. However, very few among the teachers of yoga, even if they are scholarly or formally trained, can really qualify as 'Guru'. Unlike in other spheres of learning, there are no half-way-houses here—one is either a Guru or is simply not. If one is not a Guru, and yet professes to be one, he is nothing but an imposter. For, in the words of Sir John Woodroffe—author of the classic *The Serpent Power –'trying to become a Guru without divine authority is like boarding a train without a valid ticket'.*

The debate as to the place of a Guru in a seeker's yogic quest for knowledge and freedom is a never ending one; one that pits the Eastern value of surrender against the Western notion of independence. More than anywhere else, the battle for turf between the two antithetical values rages in the mind of the East–infatuated Westerner, or the West–smitten Oriental. The significance of having an expert guide in any sphere of learning is not lost on any rational mind, since learning by trial and error, or by mere observation is demonstrably, the less efficient mode of learning. The Western mind however, feeding as it does on a spirit of questioning and rebellion, balks when asked to surrender before the supposedly complete and infallible authority of the Guru with 'eyes wide shut'. To the rational mind, this approach that in effect, purports to equate the Guru with God, amounts to intellectual slavery and in the end looks like a fresh encumbrance in 'the search for freedom'.

It goes without saying, that the West owes all its post–industrial revolution progress to its attitude of daring, rebellion and questioning—something that the Indian psyche sadly lacked in the last three centuries. At a more personal level, I can still recall the several occasions when in my school days, I entered into animated debates with the teachers and was generally prone to taking a macabre delight in vanquishing the exasperated teachers in open class-room debates. The satisfaction of one's own steadfastly held answers triumphing against all intimidating authority more than made up for the reverses at the time of annual assessments when the teachers had the opportunity to 'get even'. Again, when I was doing undergraduation in the Science faculty of the Banaras Hindu

University, I had all but lost one full academic year in bizarre circumstances, and was yet somehow able to catch up with one full year's course in Physics, Chemistry and Maths in three months of sustained self study. That I was able to accomplish this without the benefit (or distraction!) of any class room lectures and laboratory–practicals was quite a revelation to myself and the fellow students. Bunking class-room lectures for 'faster studies' at my own desk then became a habit with me in the college and in all entrance examinations in future. In hindsight, I have no reason to regret this as this strategy somehow never let me down. The values of questioning and self-help in the matters of the mind have, therefore, been as dear and familiar to me as to the average 'rebel'. And yet, I have now no hesitation in accepting that while questioning and rebellion serve a very useful purpose in the pursuit of yoga at the initial stage, the same qualities must make way for a near complete surrender of the ego along with a near-complete faith in the omniscience/omnipotence of the Guru, if the seeker's toils are to reach fruition.

Complete surrender of the ego and complete faith in the 'omniscient' Guru! Sounds untenable! Two things, however, require clarification here. Firstly, whenever one talks of perfection in the context of yoga, it is a goal forever to be approximated, yet seldom to be fully realized. The seeker need not worry about full realization since, more often than not the process of yoga takes more than a life-time to consummate and yet, showers enough bounties on the seeker at each step, to keep him more than interested all along the journey.

The second point is even more significant. As we have seen, the Guru, by definition is much more than a teacher. Before he even thinks in terms of a complete surrender to the would-be-Guru, the seeker must test the Guru a thousand times with the same tools of intellectual reasoning and questioning that he has to finally part with. For, while intellectual reasoning can never suffice or aid in measuring the true greatness of the Guru, it would generally be incisive enough to tell the chaff from the rice. In order that one gradually brings oneself to unquestioningly believe in the supposedly omniscient Guru, the Guru must really be that and nothing else. An unquestioning surrender before a guru, who was really a fraud is the worst thing that can happen to a gullible seeker. Sadly I have seen many examples of exploitative gurus and fake *diksha*s in recent times and have yet been unable to wean away the unsuspecting disciples for the fear that one has to tread carefully in the land of faith and devotion. I am however, at liberty to make use of these pages to call a spade a spade and, lest any of my readers become an easy prey to these wily 'New Age' gurus, I would mention some of the most essential and distinctive characteristics of a real Guru that one should be ever on the look out for. Briefly, these are as under:

(i) A Guru may be very erudite, semi-literate or even illiterate. Intellectual ability is of little consequence here, save that a Guru who was also scholarly, was more likely to give greater mental satisfaction and overt guidance to the disciples. Remember however, that the Guru essentially is a giver of light, not of scholastic knowledge or theological discourses, and in this sense, is more like a lamp than a book.

(ii) A Guru is invariably a *Siddha* though all *Siddhas* do not become Gurus. A *Siddha* does or does not become a Guru according to the God-Commandment or '*Adesha*'. (All *Siddhas* are in direct touch and communion with God through their open Crown Centre—*Sahasrara*—and act in strict accordance with the divine Will.)

(iii) A Guru will be positively averse to any kind of self-aggrandizement, ostentation and publicity, preferring instead to maintain a rather low profile. For this reason, he would also usually desist from an open display of miracles or *Siddhis*. *Siddhis*, however, fascinating to the supplicant, are child's play for any *Siddha*, and are in any case ranked very low down in the yoga hierarchy; something best ignored in order not to become a fixation. To the discerning eye however, most Gurus would be occasionally seen to be capable of such miracles as instant cure of serious/terminal illnesses and foretelling of impending troubles, since the welfare of the supplicants is the thing uppermost in the mind of the Guru.

(iv) The most distinguishing mark of the Guru, however, is the ability to perform *Shaktipat* or transmission of spiritual energy. The Guru is invariably, therefore, the Big Flame that can move around lighting one small candle after another without much fuss or fanfare. He has to necessarily partake the *karmic* debt of his disciples during the process of *diksha* and thereafter. And the process of *diksha* in itself is a very sacred, personal and private affair between one Guru and one deserving disciple at a given time in which karma–transference invariably takes place.

(v) Be doubly wary of the high profile, New Age guru who is likely to be intellectually gifted and logically brilliant, but who would have the all important thing missing, viz., God-realization. A *Siddha* Guru would compare to his New Age counterpart as a man, to a corpse. The man may lack manners, lack expression, lack clothes even. The corpse on the other hand, may be of good visage and anointed. Take your pick!

(vi) Since *Shaktipat*, the easiest and most powerful yoga, is all about a willing disciple running into a condescending Guru, I would try giving here a ready reckoner with thumb rules. Try them as broad hints, and develop your own intuition as the final guide:

Give-aways	Siddha Guru	New Age guru	Native guru
Speech	Terse, Cryptic	Brilliant	Loquacious
Manners	Disarming	Stand-offish	Contrived
Dress	Casual/Scant	Sophisticated	Meticulous
Gives	Peace	Titillation	Confusion
Expects	Nothing	Money, Subscription	Money
Promotes	You	Himself, Cult	Himself
Seeks	Anonymity	Publicity	Publicity
Thrives on	Scriptures	Fads, Jargon,	Wit, Superstition
Food habits	None	Elitist	Normal
Wary of	Nothing	Staleness, Criticism	Scrutiny
Ego	Absent	Massive	Inflated
Female companions	Generally none	Visible presence	Generally not disclosed
Diksha /attunement	Direct/Private /Free	Expensive, On web sites	Paid, En-masse
Sex life	Generally absent	Generally Licentious	Normal
Life style	Rudimentary	High flying	Well organized

Karma Transference

Yogi Hans Baba once told me that to give *diksha* is an onerous responsibility for the Guru, since the burden of the seeker's karmas shifts in large measure to the Guru who suffers it willingly. K. N. Rao also recounts how his own Guru, Swami Parmananda Saraswati, who was quite liberal in initiating the seekers, wore a noticeably darker countenance and suffered ill-health for some time after each *diksha*. In his book '*Ramakrishna and his Disciples*', Christopher Isherwood has a terminally ill Ramkrishna hinting to Vivekananda that the abscesses formed in his body were actually the result of supplicants' touching his body and transferring their karmas to his person. Indeed, the throat cancer that finally destroyed the physical frame of Ramakrishna is widely believed to have come from Girish Chandra Ghosh, the maverick Bengali playwright, through 'the power of attorney' he apparently wrote in favour of Ramakrishna at the saint's own insistence.

Exactly how the supremely sacrificing Guru takes on the *karmic* burden of the disciples to speed up their healing, is graphically described by Yogananda Paramahansa:

> " *The metaphysical method of physical transfer of disease is known to highly advanced yogis. A strong man may assist a weak one by helping the latter to carry a heavy load; a spiritual superman is able to minimize the physical and mental troubles of his disciples by assuming a part of their karmic burdens. Just as a rich man relinquishes some money when he pays off a large debt for his prodigal son, who is thus saved from the dire consequences of his folly, so a master willingly sacrifices a portion of his bodily wealth to lighten the misery of disciples.*
> *"By a secret yogic method, the saint unites his mind and astral vehicle with those of a suffering individual; the disease is conveyed, wholly or in part, to the yogi's fleshly form. Having harvested God on the physical field, a master is no longer concerned with his body. Though he may allow it to become diseased in order to relieve other persons, his mind, unpollutable, is not affected. He considers himself fortunate in being able to render such aid..........*
> *"A guru's work in the world is to alleviate the sorrows of mankind, whether through spiritual means or intellectual counsel or will power or physical transfer of disease... By putting on the ailments of others, a yogi can satisfy, for them, the karmic law of cause and effect".*

(Paramahansa Yogananda, *Autobiography of a Yogi*. Los Angeles: Self-Realization Fellowship, 1998)

As such, those gurus who encourage unwieldily large followings and dispense *diksha* in hoards in the midst of public ceremonies are nothing but imposters. As for the New Age gurus who peddle *diksha* through audio-visuals and websites, the less said, the better.

To Recap

Shaktipat, Mantra and Initiation

1. True yoga starts only with the awakening of the *Kundalini—shakti*. The key to quick success in yoga is in awakening the energies within, and getting them to do the 'job' for you.
2. Scriptures describe various ways in which the *Kundalini-shakti* can be awakened.
3. The safest and best way to awaken the inner energies however, is by receiving *Shaktipat* initiation from a *Siddha* Guru—preferably in the form of an energized mantra.
4. *Shaktipat*-yoga is the quintessential Yoga, containing all other yogas in their most concentrated form.
5. Only that mantra can quickly unlock the seeker's inner energies, which has been directly and individually received from a *Siddha* Guru, and is thus energized.
6. Mantras taken from any other source—from teachers, preceptors and books—are inert and largely ineffective; collective or 'electronic' *diksha* is fake initiation.
7. Mantra-repetition post initiation, makes use of sound/thought vibrations to powerfully act on the seeker's astral body—the *nadis* and *chakras*.

The Guru

8. A genuine Guru is invariably a *Siddha* though all *Siddhas* do not become Gurus.

9. The Guru is likely to be low profile; averse to publicity, self promotion and amassing of wealth for personal consumption.
10. The surest sign of a *Siddha* Guru is his proven ability to give *Shaktipat* experience whereby he is able and willing to selflessly take on the *karmic* burden of the seekers.

VIII. Reiki

'God heals and the doctor takes the fee.'

— BENJAMIN FRANKLIN

It is not very well understood, but nevertheless, is a fact of life that like disease, health is also infective. The relatively lighter spiritual methods of healing make use of a strong-willed person's mental concentration to impact and overwhelm the impressionable mental state of a sick person. However, healing that draws upon the power of the *Kundalini* or the *Holy Spirit* is deep, enduring and truly captivating. This healing transcends the constraints of time and space and prevails regardless of the severity of disease. This is the type of healing—healing through the power of the Holy Spirit—that has been demonstrated by the Perfect Ones; Krishna, Buddha and Jesus in the ancient times to Ramakrishna, Nityananda and Yogi Hans Baba more recently.

It is in the above background that I propose to take the reader towards understanding *Reiki*, the much in demand New Age art (Some would say commerce!) of spiritual healing that makes a fascinating study, irrespective of its ethical and *karmic* dimensions.

'The Universal Life Energ

The word *Reiki* literally means *universal life energy*. It refers to an esoteric, yet simple hands–on healing technique that has its origins in the ancient Indian *Tantra* System of Yoga, and that was rediscovered by Dr. Mikao Usui of Japan in late 19th century. The essence of the Reiki system of healing is transferred from a master-teacher to the student through a hierarchy of mystical initiations, much like *Shaktipat,* that in keeping with the Buddhist *Tantric* tradition, are called *'attunements'*. We have already seen how quantum physics and yoga theory both recognize energy as the substratum of all existence, and shatter the myth of 'solid matter'. Reiki then is the essential nature of the universe and the Usui method of spiritual healing, commonly known as Reiki, is but a method of fortifying ourselves with more concentrated doses of what we ourselves basically are: *universal life energy.* As a system of energy–medicine, Reiki originated in ancient India and passing through Tibet and China, went into relative oblivion before being rediscovered in the modern times by Dr. Usui. Dr. Usui is believed to have laid his hands on a medieval Buddhist manuscript *The Tantra of the Lightning Flash That Heals the Body and Illuminates the Mind.* He devised an abridged version of this seven level *Tantric* teaching to retain its essence and divided it into stages to be taught sequentially and phase-wise to the students, depending on his trust in them and their own preparedness.

Attunements

The Usui Reiki admits of three stages or Degrees. At the First Degree level, there are all together four attunements, whereas in Second and Third Degrees, there is one attunement each. Attunements are ritualistic exercises that implant the seed energy of the universal life force cutting asunder the blockages of ignorance that deny us access to the Infinite Reservoir of Energy—the source of all healing and enlightenment. Like in the *Siddha* tradition of *Shaktipat* initiation, these attunements must be received from a master-teacher who is part of the unbroken living tradition of masters of the present and past that ultimately goes back to a realized master . The Usui Reiki attunements can then be legitimately imparted only by a Reiki master who is in the direct lineage of Dr. Usui. There is one vital difference between the *Reiki* and *Shaktipat* traditions however. The *Shaktipat* tradition of *Siddhas* is much more restrictive, demanding and rarefied in that a master in the *Siddha* tradition must himself have become God-realized before being able to pass on the tradition down the line to his own disciples by way of *Shaktipat* initiation. The comparatively much watered-down Reiki tradition only requires that the master-teacher be in the direct lineage of Dr. Usui, and it is just conceivable that none in the Usui tradition, except Dr. Usui himself, was a God-realized being. If you wish to get attuned therefore, then in choosing your prospective Reiki master-teacher, you cannot afford to be as exacting and selective as in the matter of choosing a Guru for *Shaktipat* initiation. Anyone who was a reasonably decent human being and who could trace his lineage back to Dr. Usui in the matter of his own Third Degree attunement, was good enough to give you the necessary Reiki initiation.

Classically, *First Degree Reiki* consisting of four attunements in all, is given over a four day period, and the *Second Degree Reiki* that takes one day, can follow only after three months' practice of the First Degree. These days however, the trend is to compress the First and Second Degrees and give them in succession within two days. This is done ostensibly to fit into the tight schedule of prospective seekers in today's fast life, and also to give students a more palpable feel of the post-attunement experiences. Whatever the purists might say, there appears to be little harm in shortening of the duration so long as the teacher–student duo has the necessary ability and willingness to handle it. As a matter of fact, I myself received the First and Second Degrees in one single day within two hours of each other, and I don't regret it. And in about an year's time, I have followed it up by getting the Third Degree—the Master's—as my master-teacher's confidence in me grew commensurately.

Degrees and Symbols

The First Degree Reiki enables you to practise a simpler version of healing on self and others while the Second Degree gives you the necessary exposure to three Japanese Symbols that enable you to access higher powers of healing. At the practitioners' level, the First and Second Degrees together, cover all aspects you need to assimilate, so as to become adept in applying the ancient healing technique. The Third Degrcc is only for people who not only want to heal, but who wish to become master-teachers themselves. Classically, the Third Degree should be contemplated at least after three years of Reiki practice on self and hundreds of others. While the First and Second Degrees are usually learnt in a small group over the weekend, the Third Degree was intended to be an intensely private affair between a ripe student and the master-teacher in what should ideally be a life long association for both parties. As regards the four Reiki Symbols, these are given to the student on the assumption that they are not to be made public; three at the time of Second Degree attunement, and the fourth and final Symbol, at the time of attunement in the Third. The Symbols carry both form and sound, to be visualized and internally repeated like a mantra at the time of invoking Reiki for healing and allied purposes. These sacred symbols are, the *Power Symbol*, the *Emotion Symbol,* the *Distant-healing Symbol* and the *Master Symbol.* Together, the Power and Emotion Symbols make for faster healing. The Distant Symbol makes it possible for the healer to transcend limitations of time and space. (Sitting in your drawing room in Delhi you can send the Reiki across to New York, even to the past or future!) Finally, the Master Symbol enables the Reikist to become a master-teacher himself, who can then attune others.

Treatment and Cure

The generally accepted practice in Reiki treatment is to first go for whole body treatment with hand positions, so as to cover all the important organs and the endocrine glands. Only then, specific trouble-spots are picked up for more intensive treatment. Some Reikists prefer to work on the *chakra* system of the astral body, placing their hands on each of the seven *chakra* locations before zeroing in on the specific *chakras* that are suspected to give rise to particular diseases. Too much should not however, be read into the methodology since Reiki by definition is universal energy that by itself *knows* the trouble spots and flows to them automatically over a period of time. Another interesting fact is that in Reiki, the Universal Life Force is said to be *drawn* by the patient and not given by the Reikist, so that the Reikist is only a medium rather than the source, of this energy. Typically one treatment session may continue for some thing like forty-five minutes and two to three of such sessions over a week may usually suffice to cure minor/episodic disorders. Chronic diseases such as tumours, arthritis and diabetes will quite obviously, show improvement only over a longer period and in these cases Reiki gives the best (although by no means guaranteed) results in combination with other therapeutic helps such as meditation, diet discipline, Ayurveda/Homeopathy and of course, Allopathy when really needed.

In case of chronic or acute diseases however, symptoms may sometimes get worse and /or certain after-effects may appear just after treatment, about which the patient may be forewarned. This however, is likely to last for only two or three days and is part of the detoxification or purging process that is necessary for permanent and holistic cure. A running nose, frequent visits to the loo, body aches, giddiness, uneasy sensations and even vomiting may result which the patient must calmly let pass as these are sure signs of recovery. Drinking a lot of water in these conditions should bring a lot of relief, as should proper fasting and meditation. It should be taken as axiomatic that Reiki can never harm a patient, whatever be the disease or circumstances. In an odd instance however, the fast-acting Reiki can mislead doctors, specially by masking symptoms.

Reiki Possibilities

Dr. Usui had himself this to say about Reiki as a healing method:

> *"What has been transmitted is only the pacification which is called the Soothing Hand, the healing. It helps to pacify, heal and soothe, but there is much more beyond this simple technique. It does not address the activity of healing in a direct manner. It addresses it in an indirect manner by increasing the body's energy, by relaxing the tension of the body, and pacifying the upsets and imbalances."*

Notwithstanding the astronomical expenditures on treatment of diseases, every second working American is suffering from some physical ailment or chronic disease. The ratio becomes far worsened when the American population as a whole, including elders, is reckoned. Back in India, 20 percent of school-going children in New Delhi and Calcutta suffer from asthma. Due to undernourishment, greater environmental degradation and poorer living conditions in general, the Indian sub-continental population is exposed to much greater health hazards than the developed world making cancer, strokes, kidney disorders, arthritis, diabetes and osteoporosis almost epidemic. An eclectic, proactive approach to maintenance and restoration of health at the individual and societal levels is now beginning to make more and more sense, both medically and economically. Given the highly unsatisfactory results of even the most sophisticated and cost prohibitive allopathic treatments, the more natural methods of cure are called for to chip in. Reiki as part of the alternative therapy movement, has certainly demonstrated its effectiveness and versatility in recent times.

Heightened energy levels, greater inner peace and emotional highs seem to be concomitants of Reiki treatment, as they are with most successful holistic techniques, specially meditation.

My Experiences

As already mentioned, I got the First and Second Degrees within a couple of hours of each other in a single day. (It is another matter that I had by that time been meditating for last few years with *Shaktipat* initiation from a *Siddha* Guru and was probably therefore, mentally and spiritually, more up to it.) Although by this time I had become a convert to theism and was quite prepared to believe in the 'beyond and after', I still viewed Reiki suspiciously. I was virtually gambling when I rushed into Reiki. As if confirming my earlier apprehensions, I found Reiki not working at all when I first tried it on others, specially on wife, children and my mother. Although I did not need Reiki for my own meditation I, just for the sake of experimenting, used the Reiki Symbols in place of the mantra repetition once or twice. To be honest, I did find certain subtle differences in my meditation-states as soon as I invoked the Reiki Symbols, and sensed my breathing patterns change. This evidence however, was too thin to keep my interest in Reiki going. My involvement with *Shaktipat Sadhana* had already been raising a few eyebrows of late within the family, and I did not want everyone else around to believe that I was going overboard, specially as I myself had many reservations about Reiki the way it was being taught and practised these days. Things went on till I forgot all about Reiki in another six months' time. Then, a curious thing happened.

My wife has been a chronic patient of asthma all these years. When the attack comes, though not very frequently, it would not normally stop without several strong doses of cortico-steroids and salbutamol being thrust in orally and intravenously. All this was a cause of worry since we were well aware of the strong side-effects that this medication would have on her system in the long run. To add to this, I was new to the insensitive city of Delhi and was living in a make-shift house. Getting timely and reliable allopathic care was equally a problem of logistics. Just when I was beset with a whole lot of problems, came this crisis, that later on turned out to be a blessing in disguise, but that then looked very depressing. Sure enough, my wife suffered yet another of those ordinarily unmanageable attacks in the small hours of the morning with no ready allopathic assistance in sight. In the past my wife had once or twice reported some relief (which I surmised, was more psychological) when in these conditions, I had put my hand around her and silently repeated the *Gayatri mantra* myself. Quite unexpectedly, as if through a divine design, she made a request that I repeat the same process. Coincidentally, in those very months Yogi Hans Baba had come to Delhi two–three times in quick succession and my frequent touching of his feet and simply being in his presence for long hours in relative privacy had had an electrifying effect on me. Although this then appeared to be of no consequence insofar as I grappled with my wife's asthma, in hindsight all this appeared to be connected.

As I set about repeating the *Gayatri mantra* with my hands placed on wife's forehead, I suddenly recalled that I had learnt Reiki some time back, and in desperation, thought of giving it just another try. If the *Gayatri mantra*, not exactly meant for therapeutic use, could bring at least some psychological relief, then may be, the Japanese Symbols of healing also could. What happened next was nothing short of a miracle. As I practised Reiki on her, she began having strong sensations of heat and vibration in the head and chest region. In about forty-five minutes of sustained Reiki, her asthmatic attack had all but evaporated without any medication. What was left was a feeling of weakness which also vanished, as if by magic, when I repeated the same procedure in the afternoon. The transition was so dramatic and total that while she was all set for hospitalization in the morning, we were happily shopping together in one of the polluted markets of Delhi for essential purchases that very evening! After that there was no looking back. One after another, I tried Reiki on my children, close friends and even some office colleagues. Invariably, Reiki made a powerful impression on all though healing took different detours in each case, sometimes becoming visible immediately after a session, sometimes working silently at deeper levels to remove blockages, even occasioning temporary after-effects in isolated cases as part of the purging process.

I then began to suspect that the fast-acting healing influences that had started simply flowing through my hands in abundance at my slightest will, were not Reiki entirely as taught to me, but equally, were inspired by the powerful *Shaktipat* experiences that I had been blessed with by Yogi Hans Baba. Around this time only, I started having distinct *Kundalini* experiences every time I sat either for mantra repetition or for Reiki healing. Typically, when I gave Reiki to some one, I would first myself go through a whole range of sensations (which I subsequently began to consciously internalize) and wait for them to subside before I could invoke Reiki for healing. Since no Reiki expert (including my own master-teacher in whom I vainly confided without his having any clue), insofar as I know, treated his patient in this highly unusual manner, I had reason to conclude that the healing that took place through my medium was as much Hans Baba's blessing to the patient (second hand!) as it was Reiki. Small miracles then became routine in my household as my wife, suffering a headache, my children, down with viral fever, would come to me to be offered Reiki, and in a matter of hours rather than days, feel not only cured, but unusually energetic. And then came the miracle of all miracles!

The Yoga/Reiki inspired miracles that would often catch me off-guard, were increasing by the day and taking me deeper and deeper into God faith and meditation, even as my external problems showed no signs of relenting. Rajiv, my brother-in-law and now an American citizen, was then on a short trip to India and staying with us. A rationally inclined multinational executive, he watched the fascinating changes occurring in and around me with keen interest. By the time he decided to see Yogi Hans Baba along with me, he was so much impressed as to seek and get spiritual initiation from the great Guru. Meanwhile I rang up my mother at Patna to tell all that was happening and she sounded more concerned than excited that I was going 'the yogi way'. Then one day, even as I and Rajiv were chatting, there came the ring at the dead of night. My mother it was, anxious and weeping, who told me that our dear *mausi* (mother's sister) was in the ICU at the small town of Giridih with a protracted and near fatal bout of asthma. She informed that doctors attending on her had all but given up hope. Mother said that she had been herself frantically praying to Yogi Hans Baba, and pleaded that I use Reiki to save her if possible. My first internal reaction was one of concern for my mother's own well being, for she was herself not in the best of health those days. This distressing news, if it grew any worse, could be just too much for her as well.

I was not a professional healer anyway, and with this bewildering turn of events, I was at my wit's end. Till then I had not practised distant healing on anyone, let alone on someone who was actually dying or even dead by the time I tried to do something. Initially, I thought of trying Reiki on my mother, rather than my aunt partly because after all, my mother came first, and also because I wanted to try the healing energy on a living rather than a nearly lost cause. But God probably willed it otherwise, and on some counselling by Rajiv and my wife, I sat in deep meditation sending Reiki across to my aunt, fighting for her life in the ICU of a non-descript government hospital in Bihar some 1500 kms. away. The next hour of Reiki and meditation was literally mind blowing; it threw up such strong vibrations together with an array of experiences that, sitting in the lotus posture, I could only awe and marvel. It was as if the piece of paper on which Reiki Symbols and the healing message were inscribed had come alive. After an hour-long encounter with the 'supernormal', I was thoroughly exhausted and yet delighted. For, intuitively I knew that my aunt had been saved by God's inscrutable Will. As I heard another long distance call coming (from my mother obviously) I, still meditating, asked Rajiv to attend the call and tell mother that '*aunt had been saved*'. It came as no big surprise to me the next day when mother, by this time having reached the Giridih hospital from Jamshedpur, rang up again and 'broke' the good news that aunt had indeed recovered dramatically. As was expected, going by Benjamin Franklin's quote, *'God healed and the doctors took the fee'*.

Reiki—A Karmic Trap?

By this time I was elated at the 'Midas touch' I had come to acquire thanks to the Universal Life Force and the blessings of my Christ like Guru. I thought I could use it responsibly, yet extensively to cure a great many suffering people—friends, relatives and colleagues. Quickly however, the bubble of excitement was to nearly burst. Soon after, I was to have my mandatory meeting with 'X', the astrologer friend. Readers would recall that it was 'X' whose prognostication had initially made me turn towards meditation and Hans Baba. A most noble person, he also is well read on scriptures. Not surprisingly therefore, I value his opinions though we do not necessarily end up agreeing on everything. I expected my discoveries in Reiki healing to come to him as a pleasant surprise. Instead it was my turn to be surprised. He told me rather matter-of-factly that he already knew enough about the near miraculous healing powers of Reiki, but did not think too highly of it because of the *karmic* considerations involved. What transpired during the thought–provoking discussions was essentially this:

Reiki is essentially an offshoot of the Indian Tantric

tradition (no arguments there). 'The Westerners (basically Americans via the Japanese) who, for all their intellectual brilliance, do not have a grounding in the Hindu philosophy, are generally unable to fully appreciate the subtleties of the invisibly, yet inexorably operating law of karma that is pivotal to a true understanding of Yoga, and that therefore cannot be just wished away. In the Yoga tradition, Tantric practices, specially of the Vama and/or ritualistic variety, though effective in bringing psychic abilities and short term gains, are generally not encouraged as means of deliverance. For, the Tantric practices represent a bye-pass that does not address the root cause of all suffering—the burden of karmas—and that therefore, necessarily brings a karmic backlash even as it seems to remove suffering in the short run. Shiva and Shakti are the active female and static male principles of Creation, representing polarities in the human body. The human condition of felt inadequacies and a fractured sensibility is the consequence of this schism. Yoga heals completely and makes man 'whole' because it ultimately reunites the awakened and rising feminine principle with the static masculine principle (the immutable God head) in the cerebral crown centre (Sahasrara). *Looking from a different angle, Shakti is Power while Shiva represents Purity. Use of Power by one who has become Pure (an illumined yogi) has the necessary God–sanction to bring about permanent healing or Yoga in mankind removing all karmic fetters. Tantra on the other hand, as practised by the majority, attempts to use Shakti without a commensurate accomplishment of Shiva, and therefore, necessarily ends up as a vicious circle in which the karmically engendered human suffering can be postponed or transferred from one to the other without being obliterated in any manner. Not surprisingly therefore, it is seen that most Tantrics meet a violent end and, in any case, have an unhappy family life.*

The practical implications of this rather esoteric and frightening account of *Tantra*, for a Reiki practitioner is that, regardless of what the Western theorists have to say of the *Universal Life Energy* using the Reikist as a mere medium, the fact according to this theory, is that the healer, unknowingly absorbs the patient's karmas and is therefore bound to commensurately suffer himself and regress as he heals. The commonsense argument that thousands of Reikist are now successfully practising healing and even making commercial gains out of it without seeming to suffer in any manner, cannot be of much value in this scheme of things. For, as scriptures tell us, the karmas that man has accumulated in past many lives and is accumulating even now, are to be not necessarily exhausted in the current life. As Lord Krishna tells Arjuna in Gita, *we have been born before hundreds of times and are likely to be born over and over again, before all our karmas can be exhausted.* Even within this life cycle, who can say for sure that the Reiki practitioners healing on a large commercial scale will not suffer the *karmic* consequences? It is to be remembered that physical diseases are but one of the many variations of suffering that negative karmas occasion. In a culture that feeds on false glitter and make–believe, you need to be almost clairvoyant to see people as they really are. Look around carefully, and you might find that behind the masks of the rich and the famous, lies a broken marriage, a departed son, a estranged daughter and above all, a restless soul!

I returned much more subdued, but still not fully convinced. Then I learnt of another person, a close relative of one of my subordinates who had had much the same experiences of the *Kundalini* and Reiki healing as me, and who now had concluded that in Reiki healing, regardless of what the Reiki expert says, energy that heals actually depletes you. Still not fully convinced, I phoned up K. N. Rao on the subject who confirmed that Reiki healing indeed had a *karmic* angle to it. (When I last met Rao, he explained that Reiki was but a milder form of *Shaktipat* with this crucial difference that whereas a *Siddha* had the necessary spiritual strength to withstand the *karmic* backlash, the run-of-the-mill Reikist didn't!) Honestly, I am not entirly convinced on whatever Rao had to say about Reiki, but coming from a spiritualist of his standing, I took it with the seriousness it deserved. Finally I put the question to Hans Baba during his next visit to Delhi. *Siddhas* however, are marked more by their reticence and laconic comments than by their loquacity. His cryptic comments could be interpreted either way given the infirmities of our limited knowing faculties. Even then, I could tentatively gather from whatever he said that karma did, in some way or the other, trail the Reikist whenever he took to healing. As regards the stand of notable Western Reiki scholars on the subject, it is well articulated and need not be repeated. In nutshell, it is that since Reiki is Universal Energy acting through the Reikist as its medium, it does not in any way deplete the Reikists. That on the other hand, the Reikist is himself healed somewhat everytime he uses Reiki, becoming himself cleansed of blockages and negativity in the process.

That the New Age theorists are not absolutely true in this regard appears certain to me. For, spiritual healing is not quite the same as more 'earthly' modes of treatment such as Allopathy and Homeopathy. By their own admission, Reiki is God's Energy, *not belonging to you.* The very idea of claiming to be acting as a *mere agent of God* in this transfer of healing energy and yet pocketing a healthy brokerage, appears repulsive to me. It leaves me convinced that these merchants of God's Grace are bound to suffer the consequences at some point of time. The pros and cons of undertaking Reiki healing on purely altruistic considerations or by charging the costs only, is an altogether different matter on which I am myself undecided as yet. My advice to the reader therefore, would then be to tread the golden middle path. Do learn Reiki (First and Second Degrees) and do it sooner than later. Confine your treatment sessions however, to your family and follow it up with lots of meditation. If it sounds somewhat selfish, it should not. For, you can always encourage others to learn Reiki themselves and tell them honestly about your own experiences. Self help is after all the best help, and there are probably any number of other less mysterious ways of doing charity. If you still needed any convincing, let me tell you this. After the frenzied rounds of healing, I did on an odd occasion feel down and fatigued, for whatever reason. And call it coincidence, call it Providence; I suffered two successive fractures of my little finger of the left hand in rather bizarre circumstances (*left hand Tantra*, did they say?) just after that which took four months to heal!

To Recap

1. Reiki is an esoteric hands-on healing technique that uses the universal life energy.
2. It has its origins in the ancient Tantra tradition of yoga; it was nonetheless rediscovered by Dr. Mikao Usui, a 19th century Japanese Buddhist.
3. Reiki initiation or 'attunement' comprises the First and Second Degrees for healing and a Third and final Degree for the healer to himself become a master-teacher.
4. Attunements are ritualistic exercises that implant the seed energy of the universal life force in such way as to remove blockages that impede our access to the infinite pool of the healing life energy.
5. At the First Degree level, there are four attunements in all, whereas at the Second and the Third, there is one attunement each.
6. The First Degree enables one to practise a simpler version of healing, while the Second gives exposure to

three Japanese Symbols that enhance healing ability. The Third Degree gives access to the fourth and final Master Symbol

7. Symbols are given to the seeker on the understanding that these are not to be divulged.
8. The Reiki treatment is fast acting and invariably efficacious regardless of the disease, although it is not a cure–all and works best in combination with other natural therapeutic techniques, such as the Ayurveda and Homeopathy.
9. The 'official' view of the Reiki School is that the Reikist is not the healer but merely a vehicle of the healing energy who thus stands to only gain in course of giving Reiki.
10. This view is however, contested by some Yoga scholars who, emphasizing the inviolability of karma save at the hands of a *Siddha*, see the Reikist invisibly suffering a karmic backlash each time he heals.
11. Regardless of its hard-to-prove karmic dimension, the money making aspect of this essentially spiritual discipline is something that must be detrimental to the Reiki mercenaries in the long run.

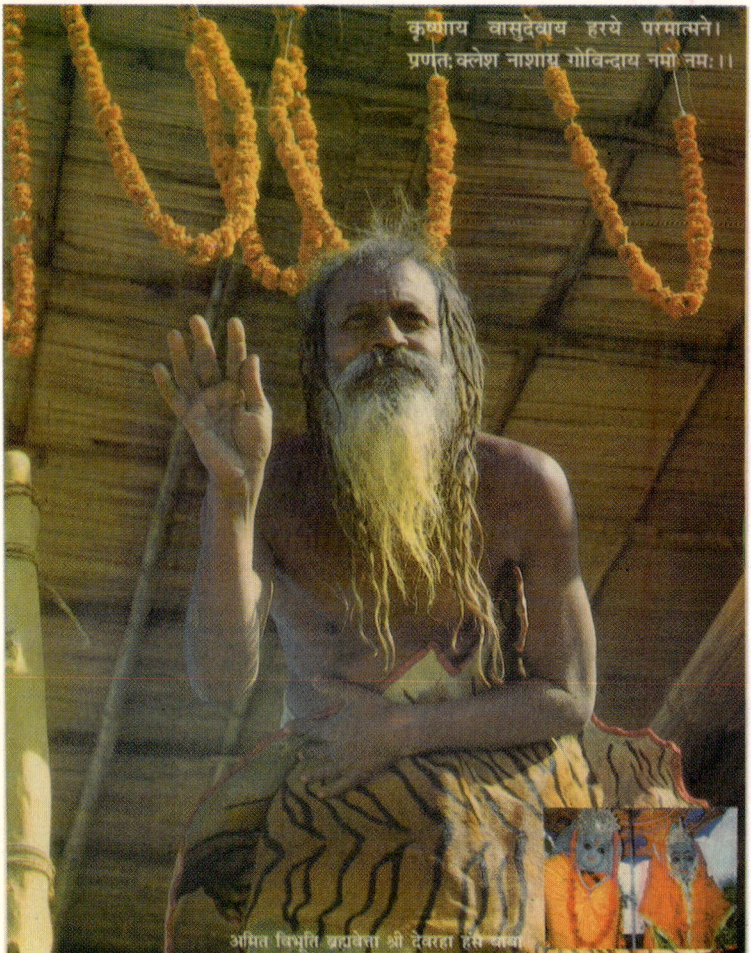
कृष्णाय वासुदेवाय हरये परमात्मने।
प्रणतः क्लेश नाशाय गोविन्दाय नमो नमः।।
अमित विभूति ब्रह्मवेत्ता श्री देवरहा हंस बाबा

छायाकार : आर. के. स्टूडियो

माघ मेला 1997 प्रयाग (इलाहाबाद) के शुभ अवसर पर भक्तों को आशीर्वाद देते हुए

IX. Yogi Hans Baba

"To know the universe itself as a road,
as many roads,
as roads for travelling Souls."

—WALT WHITMAN

In the preceding chapter, I have time and again used the word '*Siddha*' to describe the illumined yogis who have acquired complete control over nature and the self. I have also described how blessings of an illumined one, specially in the form of *Shaktipat* initiation by him, can spark off a self-propelled, self-sufficient yoga in the seeker that feeds on his own latent *Kundalini*-energies and is deeply fulfilling. Readers should not go to the pessimistic extreme of believing that there cannot be any yoga practice in the absence of a *Siddha* Guru. The yoga tradition does underline the importance of becoming a 'twice born' (*dvija*) by getting a second birth in the form of *diksha* from a *Siddha* Guru. The ground reality however, is that *Siddhas* are the rarest of rare beings, not to be easily found. Even if you run into a man of God by any chance, it is that much more unlikely that you would ever recognize his greatness at first sight. For, these yogis are usually men of few words and as a rule, do not like to talk of themselves, unlike worldly people. To make things look even more dismal, these yogis are often very selective and miserly in the matter of dispensing *diksha* since they have very high standards for their discipleship that are not easily met by lesser mortals. In his books, K. N. Rao has spoken about a number of such *Siddhas* who spiritually initiated only one disciple each in their life time, or none at all, urging visitors instead, to concentrate on *bhajans* (devotional songs) and *bhakti* (devotion) as means of deliverance.

Since the Divine Intelligence did not intend fulfillment to become the preserve of a select few, it is clear that *diksha* is a desirable, not essential feature of yoga. Regular practice of select physical *asanas,* meditation with the aid of a suitable hymn chosen on astrological and other relevant considerations, practising charity and devotion, and moderate habits including a predominantly vegetarian diet, can over a period, surely take one to such heights of yoga as to bring sufficient healing of the body, mind and spirit. There is no denying however, that *Shaktipat* initiation is the escalator route to yoga that saves you the trouble of climbing stairs. The correct way to practise yoga therefore is to continue faithfully practising all other types of yoga without despairing for the elusive Guru and, in the midst of all yogic practices, just remain alert to the possibility of some day, somewhere finding the Guru. My own experience suggests that getting a *Siddha* Guru is never a lottery, but a matter of Divine Design; a momentous event in the life of a seeker that can be made a reality and brought closer in time by going through the preparatory stages of yoga with confidence and optimism.

Fortunately, not all *Siddhas* are so tight-fisted in the matter of blessing supplicants with *diksha.* And even more fortunately, these *Siddhas*, following instructions received directly from God (*Adesha*) through their open 'crown' centre, are to be occasionally found in the hustle and bustle of city life, far removed from the remote, unseen caves of the high mountains that seem to be their natural habitat. These yogis, though still very much averse to publicity and commercialism of any manner, allow visitors to approach them in their low–key *ashrams* or at makeshift hutments at places they visit. These rare Siddhas give *Shaktipat* experiences to thousands and thousands of supplicants even though it *karmically* entails a great personal suffering for them. The guiding philosophy behind granting of *diksha* with many relaxations to the many rather than the few is that it would after all do 'some' good to 'many', even as it does 'much' good to 'a few'. It is not however advisable for a seeker to ask for spiritual initiation without a certain degree of commitment to the yoga way of life. The key to successful meditation through *diksha* is to gradually rise above too much identifying with materialistic pleasures and allowing the higher truths the necessary space to gradually emerge from the background.

The Enigma

Lest the reader began to believe that such men of God were long lost (could not survive our tough times?) or merely a figment of imagination, I would now proceed to describe one such living saint who is still amongst us and who has illumined the lives of lakhs of devotees like me. It is none other than Hans Baba about whom I have spoken earlier. My association with him is a relatively recent one dating back to 1997. However, even the short period of knowing him has been deeply fulfilling and has enabled me to make such progress in yoga as was perhaps not possible otherwise in many life-times. My getting to know Hans Baba was rather fortuitous.

I have a close friend whom I know to be somewhat psychic from his early days, and who often dabbled in mystical practices without the required preparedness of body and spirit, till he finally got into trouble. The onset of my friend's troubles became the precipitate reason for my meeting Hans Baba. It so happened that this friend, during his practising of austerities, went a little overboard and that resulted in a violent, uncontrolled rising of the 'serpent force' of *Kundalini* that started playing havoc with his mind and body. The bizarre behavioural symptoms that followed, in the absence of a Guru and his Grace to fall back upon, soon assumed such distressing proportions that the person was all but branded a schizophrenic, to be duly put under a psychiatrist's diagnostic and medicinal care. When the anxious relatives contacted me, I got his birth horoscope analysed by my astrologer friend, 'X', with whom those days I used to often converse on the finer points of astrology, Hinduism and yoga theory for long hours. It was assured that nothing catastrophic was likely and all allopathic drugs were stopped at his behest since according to him, it was a case of an abrupt rising of the *Kundalini*, rather than any sort of aberration. (It is instances such as these which show the true worth of genuine astrological counsel.) Instead it was advised that we take the 'patient' to one Hans Baba who was the chief disciple of the departed Devraha Baba, and who had within a very short time made such a huge Jesus like impact on thousands of suffering devotees with his divine healing powers as to occasion K. N. Rao's biography of him—'*Divine Love and Miracles of Yogi Hans Baba*'. Destiny was playing its own funny little game, since this 'saint on wheels' did not allow us to take the trouble of going all the way to his Vindhyachal *ashram*. Shortly, he came on a low-key visit to Patna enabling the suffering friend and his family to approach him sooner rather than later. Some members of my own family also accompanied them, and what happened next was—what else, but pure miracle! The saint, scantily clad and serenely seated on his raised wooden platform on the Ganga bank, not only permanently cured my friend of all his problems, but while doing so, took him through a whole range of *Kundalini* experiences that were tantalizingly close to the state of *Savikalpa Samadhi*, described in the scriptures. The 'poor' chap went through a whole range of gyrating motions of the upper torso (*kriyas*) that made him toss and whirl like a spinning top. Visions of dazzling inner lights and Baba's own resplendent face filled the closed eyes of my entranced friend. When he was ushered back into our 'world of illusion' by Baba himself, he could clearly see a sparkling aura around Baba's beaming face even with eyes wide open.

I was not very enthusiastic about seeing the Baba at the

beginning, and therefore, had excused myself from the trip. But when I learnt of what all had transpired in the visit from the friend and my own family members, I got interested. The next day, I duly went to see the saint, only to be somewhat disappointed to see a huge crowd gathered around him that made it virtually impossible for him to pay attention to anyone. My disappointment however, soon turned into a pleasant surprise when, at my turn, Baba took unusual interest in me, had some very affectionate words to say, and never let me feel that I was seeing him for the first time. It is only in hindsight that I can say with confidence that, with such omniscient yogis, one can never be too sure whether one was meeting them for the first or the nth time. In *Bhagavad Gita*, Krishna tells Arjuna, *"I and you have both been born umpteen times, but the difference is that I remember each of my births, while you (under the veil of Maya) have forgotten yours"*(4:5). I went to the Baba again after a couple of days and was again picked out by him from the crowd, this time with an unusually insistent 'request' (I was still not prepared to accept any of his wishes as commands) that I come to see him at his Vindhyachal *ashram* on *Guru-Purnima* that was shortly approaching. (In the Indian tradition, *Guru-Purnima* is the spiritually significant full moon day some time in the rainy season when all devotees travel to be with their Gurus and receive their blessings.) The restive crowd was thirsting for so much as a casual glance or a word of blessing/ instruction from the Godman, and here I was, evasive and recalcitrant, telling him instead that I could think of coming to him only when he visited Patna or a convenient place nearby in future! Not irritated in the least, Baba was yet emphatic that I should see him in Vindhyachal even as I 'knew' that this was not possible.

What happened next was another small miracle, of an unpleasant kind though. Baba soon came to Gaya which is only a two hour-journey from Patna. Here was the chance to see Baba once again the way I had intended rather than as Baba wished (foresaw?). Confidently I went to the railway station next day after duly ascertaining (I was a railway officer after all !) that the train was starting right time. There was this small problem though, as it turned out, in that the train's scheduled departure time had, very unusually, been advanced by 15 minutes so that by the time I reached the station, the train had left. (It is another matter that it was one in a hundred chance at any given time that this notorious Patna-Gaya passenger train would start punctually!) Disappointed I nonetheless, boarded the same train the next day, and this time the same train duly took off two hours late. After about an hour's journey however, the rarest of rare things happened. The train engine failed between two stations with a replacement engine not within sight for another six hours. Irritated and exhausted, I figured out that now I could not possibly continue on this jinxed ride as I had no plans or arrangements to stay at Gaya overnight. However, returning home was also not that easy a proposition since the ill-fated train was stranded in mid-section. In the end, I decided to trudge my way back along the tracks for 9 kms. under heavy rains. The ordeal was not complete without my catching an auto-rickshaw, then a bus, then a cycle rickshaw on my way back, before I had exhausted my 'little bad karma' of having tried to defy the biddings of a man of God. Although *Guru-Purnima* had passed by, it was not long thereafter before I, chastened and wiser, duly visited the Vindhyachal *ashram*. Since then I have learnt about many similar incidents when devotees have tried to deviate from Baba's plans set for them, and have suffered for that.

From then onwards, my association with Baba became deeper and deeper. My *diksha* followed soon after and my visits to him became more frequent. Then I began aspiring for the *Shaktipat*-triggered 'inner flames' *(jyoti)* that Baba shows many a devotee with eyes closed, and that somehow refused to come to me despite Baba's ministration. The stalemate continued for another two years or so, and Baba once voiced his concern much to my sadness. Just when I had got used to being the 'unfit one', I suddenly started experiencing it and much more as the 'serpent power'(*Kundalini* energy) got awakened under Baba's divine spell.

I do not wish to recount my own 'supernormal' experiences in these pages, for they are too personal, and in any case the reader has had enough of it in the earlier chapters. Stories of Baba having brought the dead alive, controlled rains and hailstorms, given sight to the blind and a sprightly walk to the lame, are legion. True to the tendency among human beings in general and 'blind' devotees in particular, some of these stories must be exaggerated and become part of folklore without the due exercise of caution. It is now irrefutable however that roughly over a period of last ten years, thousands and thousands of supplicants have had their physical disabilities either fully removed or substantially mitigated by Baba's Grace. That there could be an equal or bigger number of visitors who were not similarly rewarded, need not be disputed. For, the *law of karma* ultimately prevails, in which the seer's role is that of an interceder between God and the devotee. In any such instance of miracle healing, the devotee's degree of faith and surrender to God Will necessarily plays a part (remember the placebo effect?) though the yogi's divine influence is paramount. K. N. Rao's biography of Hans Baba documents numerous well researched instances of such healings by Baba during his Delhi sojourn in 1994. By his own account, *Rao then witnessed no fewer than 3000 miracle–healings* during Baba's Delhi–stay. It was here that Amrita Pritam got healed. She herself gives a moving account of her experience thus:

> *"That evening I and Imroz went to see Hans Baba. A* machan *had been prepared for him there. And below on the cleaned ground many people were sitting whom he was blessing.*

Very lean body and brownish, but it appeared that those who looked at him, got transfixed. That someone's face be so lustrously blossoming seemed to be an experience in a physical way and something supernormal. His smiling face was weaving magic spells.

He told me, "close your eyes". I closed my eyes and he asked me, "Have you experienced anything from your head to toe."

Sparks of electricity had entered my body. Therefore, when I said "yes", tears rolled down my eyes. He then asked me, "Have you seen anything". I had seen nothing, so I kept silent. ....But that night, I saw in my dream a very big forest and Hans Baba singing alone there and dancing too.... and then I saw him holding in his hand a yard long bunch of grapes .... and he dancing with those grapes in his hand.

In such a stupor–like condition next few days rolled by. I felt that in the inner consciousness many atoms of the super conscious lie somnolent which get awakened after meeting someone....

I told him about my dream.... he again laughed and said, "sit in front of me". I was standing and knew that I would not be able to sit down because of the pain in my left knee which is chronic. When I told him about it, he said "there would be no pain. Sit down". It being his instruction, I sat down. I was suffering, I kept quite. He said, "leave your pain here". ....

The heaviness I have been experiencing from my waist to the knees, was still persisting. I therefore said, "There is pain, Baba. This part of my body is as though in knots"....
He then looked skyward and said, raising his hand in blessing, "I am now doing shakti-paat. Tell me what you are feeling."

I was puzzled, I looked at my knees. There was no pain....."

(In the Punjabi monthly "Nagmani" edited by Amrita Pritam)

How would the medical mainstream react to Baba's therapeutic feats? Sample this—

> *"I have also encountered people who got no relief for their ailments. But that is not puzzling. What is puzzling is the fact that medically incurable ailments showed relief. As if the Baba manipulated the subtle cosmic powers through a remote control to cause healing. No medical methods can make a patient of crippling cardiomyopathy to walk unrestrained for two hours without the slightest sign of distress. This happened in my very presence to a lady who could not take ten paces at a stretch without pausing for breath. Another young man started hearing through his left ear which had suffered apparently irreparable damage from an injury sustained early in his childhood. He had been declared medically incurable."*

Dr. K.S. Charak,
Head of Surgery Department,
Indira Gandhi ESI Hospital, Delhi

On my part, I wish to describe two poignant instances of Baba's *'Leela'* (divine play)that I enjoy most. The first instance relates to one Bhola Babu, a pious man and retired government employee from Patna who has become so much devoted to Baba that he now spends most of his time at the Vindhyachal *ashram* at his feet, offering his services in the cause of the impressive Radha-Krishna temple that is coming up within the *ashram* premises. The *ashram* is set inside thick jungles, and it so happened one midnight that poor Bhola Babu was bitten by a scorpion. Screaming in pain, the old man could do only one thing—jump out of the bed, rush to Baba and fall on his feet crying incessantly all the while, all in one motion. Baba, ever the picture of calmness, said some comforting words to the hapless victim. He then proceeded to tap the *machan* two–three times and asked the poor man how he felt now. Viola! The excruciating pain had largely left his body in seconds, although it continued with the same ferocity in his affected arm. Baba tapped the *machan* again, and repeated the same question. God! The pain had disappeared from the rest of the arm, although it was still there with all its sting in the palm of the hand. Baba tapped the *machan* a third time, and Bhola Babu, still in agony, responded by informing that the pain had now got confined to the little finger of the palm where the bite had taken place. At this stage Baba asked the victim to brave the remaining pain, informing him of the *karmic* background of the whole event that went back not only to his own past birth, but also involved the regressive birth cycle of his adversary of this and previous lives. Bhola Babu, came the revelation, had become the cause of a lot of suffering to one person in his past life and had thereby incurred bad karma. Since this gentleman himself was no paragon of virtue, he was born in this life as a black scorpion, intent on taking revenge from his adversary of past life in the running trans–life, trans-species feud. As soon as the opportunity presented itself, the man-turned scorpion had taken revenge! As the pain subsided, Bhola Babu was instructed to go back to his bed, but only after getting rid of the ferocious scorpion that was "still hiding in the bed sheets". Sure enough, the culprit in question—a giant sized scorpion whose bite should have killed—was discovered by disciples and gingerly carried away to the safety of the jungles according to Baba's instructions.

If the above tale, every inch true since I personally know Bhola Babu and have even seen the scar on his affected finger, is reminiscent of the saga of Shirdi's Sai Baba, so be it. Strange are the ways of all Godmen, and the second tale that I am going to recount now is no less strange. It was probably in 1998 that a white middle aged American arrived at Baba's *ashram* and spoke to him with the help of an interpreter who just about passed muster (the omniscient Baba himself is semi-literate, insofar as formal learning goes). The Westerner was spiritually inclined and had somehow come to see Baba after a twenty years' relentless globe-trotting in search for the 'meaning of life'. On being asked about his wish, he wanted to know or better still 'see' what he was like in his previous birth. Baba granted his unusual request and for a considerable time thereafter, the visitor, with eyes closed in veneration, 'saw' his own childhood form of the past life. He was then a prankster living near the Ganges and used to teasing the sages who sat on the bank deep in meditation. As the boy's pranks became nastier and nastier, one day one of the sages solemnly told him that even as he was having fun at the expense of men of God in that life, he was destined to be born far away from those pious surroundings and sages in his next life, and was doomed to pine for the heavenly company that he did not value in the current life. The foreigner's trance however did not stop at the concluding scene of his previous life. Instead he now began 'seeing' the forms of Hans Baba and his own self dancing in delight alongside the dallying pair of Krishna and Goddess Radha! Baba kept mum as tears of gratitude and ecstasy overcame the American. It was not the reticent Baba, but the American himself who told others around about his experiences under Baba's spell, after gathering his wits. On his way back, the happy and enlightened Westerner readily wrote down his name and address for the benefit of *ashram*-indwellers.

Guru 'finds' the disciple

Time and again, I have stressed that beginners desirous of *Shaktipat-yoga,* must not be too obsessed or impatient in their search for the *Siddha* Guru. How destiny unfolds itself, and how the Guru himself 'spots' the right disciple at the right time, is underlined by one incident involving Hans Baba and a former Head of Department of Paediatrics at Darbhanga Medical College, Bihar who incidentally happens to be closely related to me.

Dr. Bhola Nayak, a very reputed doctor, had been interested in yoga for the last few years. It was only recently however, that he seriously took to meditation. His meditation practices however, were not giving him full satisfaction since, by his own admission, he was torn from within by the conflicting pulls of whether or not to seek a Guru. Like many others, he uncertainly reasoned with himself, that total surrender before a Guru who was 'just another mortal', amounted to intellectual slavery. Yet, all Hindu scriptures that he greatly respected, were unanimous that the Guru is God personified for the seeker. A doctor–colleague of his, whose insight I must admire, then once told him not to loose his sleep over the issue and instead, carry on his meditation, since 'when he was ripe enough, the Guru would Himself pluck him.' Now Dr. Nayak is a busy medical practitioner even after retirement, who normally can ill afford to skip his clinic for even one day. There was no conceivable way, he could get a Guru by travelling around, even if he had the will. That he had no such definite inclination, made it virtually impossible.

It so happened that under family–pressure, he agreed to come to Delhi precisely for one day, in order to attend a function in Delhi. That two of his married daughters were staying in Delhi was a bonus. Once in Delhi, he started talking to me about his meditation, and wondered where, if at all, he could find the right guru, in the midst of his tight schedule. The topic was soon forgotten as he prepared to leave by the evening train. I think, it was March, 1999. Just then, came the news of a great political turmoil in Bihar, in the aftermath of change of government. Arson and violence broke out, and all train–services between Delhi and Bihar got diverted / disrupted. Since a skeleton train–service between Delhi and

Bihar was somehow being kept up by the railway authorities, I kept trying, as a railway officer, to somehow send Dr. Nayak back to Bihar by some train or the other. As he was advised against flying, he became desperate as message came of the gathering chaos at his busy Darbhanga clinic. Over the next five days, every single train by which I intended to book and dispatch him, got cancelled at the last moment. There was a sombre atmosphere in my drawing room with me at my wit's end, and the doctor marooned and helpless.

At that instant, out of the blue, came this long distance call that Hans Baba was, for the next day-and–a-half, available in Delhi. In a flash, it occurred to me that all this apparent chaos signalled, in our context, only one thing; that the doubting, yet deserving doctor was destined to be blessed by Hans Baba during that nightmarish visit, after some *karmic* suffering. I told this much to him, and when he showed an inclination, I drove him to Baba's place next morning. Once there, all his initial skepticism and professional pride could not prevent him from becoming spell-bound and getting spiritually initiated by Baba. His *diksha* over, all train services got miraculously restored that very evening and he left by the train of his choice. Thus it was, that the Guru truly 'found out' his ripe disciple against all odds. Ever since, the doctor has been making impressive spiritual progress back home.

Paravani

True to the scriptural description, Baba speaks his spiritually pregnant *paravani* or divine song in 'strands and pearls'. To the first timer, this appears to be all jumbled up, meaningless and even irritating. Only the discerning and the faithful among the men around however, know that this *paravani,* flowing divinely from his tongue, contains some of the greatest healing powers and prophecies that human beings would come across in modern times. I am here tempted to quote K. N. Rao again, who more than anyone else, is competent to make meaning out of the jigsaw puzzles that

Baba's utterances often are—

> *"In Delhi, I had taken to Baba most of those friends who had been taking astrological predictions from me for many years. I knew them, their problems, their ambitions, their agonies and their past, even if sordid. The moment they went to Baba, the* vani *that emerged described their problems exactly, both their agony and their ambitions. I have never seen a more dazzling demonstration of instantaneous prophecy. .... "*

(*Divine Love and Miracles of Yogi Hans Baba*: K.N. Rao)

A *Siddha*

Patanjali's *Yoga Sutra* makes an apt description of the state of attainment of a *Siddha* or the perfected yogi. A *Siddha* is one who has complete control over the forces of the universe, and over his inner universe. Simply put, a *Siddha* is one who has become one with God by realizing *Nirvikalpa Samadhi* or the state of changeless God-consciousness. *Vikalpa* literally means difference or non-identity. The lower state of *Savikalpa Samadhi* is the state of God-consciousness with difference; *Nirvikalpa* is the God consciousness state without duality. In *Savikalpa* state, the seeker directly perceives God, but with a thin veil of separation. In *Nirvikalpa*, he becomes totally merged in God to loose his identity and become the Spirit. In *Savikalpa* state, the seeker cannot retain his Cosmic Consciousness save in the unstable trance state. In the highest state of *Nirvikalpa* however, the seeker, now become *Siddha*, becomes permanently established in the Cosmic Consciousness. He may then freely engage in worldly activities without any impairment of God-consciousness. It is for this reason that Hans Baba, fully and irreversibly established in *nirvikalpa samadhi*, is able to interact with so many worldly people day-in and day-out, and yet does not loose his own purity one bit.

The Early Days

There can be some debate on whether the sinners really 'have no future', specially in this age of materialism when, to quote W.B. Yeats, *"the best lack all conviction and the worst are full of passionate intensity"*. There can be little doubt however, that saints 'have no past', transcend as they do all limitations of time, space and that veil of ignorance—*maya.* Outwardly, all *Siddhas* are like us but in truth they are the disembodied Holy Spirit 'made flesh' by God's Will to help us rise above body-consciousness and become established in Yoga. *Siddhas* themselves instruct seekers to live in and make the most of the all important present, without worrying about the dead past and the uncertain future. For this reason, in my several long and fruitful meetings with Hans Baba I have never once broached the delicate subject of Baba's past, and instead remained satisfied with whatever was gathered of it from Baba's other noted devotees. Inquisitiveness as to his antecedents—native place,parents, age and caste—is hardly in order, since in the *Sanyasa* tradition that Baba symbolizes, there is no room for the buried past. A reasonably reliable account of Baba's early days, as pieced together by journalists and scholars in course of sundry conversations, goes like this.

Very early in his life, Hans Baba became restless in his search for God. He set out wandering probably in some part of Eastern Uttar Pradesh near his native place, till in desperation he tried to end his 'Godless existence' by throwing himself in a dry well. The story goes that at that instant, Saraswati, Goddess of wisdom made a cosmic manifestation and instructed the rescued Hans to approach Devraha Baba. The legendary seer of modern times was then possibly camping on the banks of the Ganga river in the holy city of Prayaga (Allahabad). The young seeker duly went to have the yogi's *darshana* and was immediately spotted by the saint to be quickly made his disciple. It was Devraha Baba who christened the would-be yogi as 'Hans', the word literally standing for a swan and figuratively meaning the soul. A few of his initiated disciples used to permanently stay with Devraha Baba and practise *Sadhana* unobtrusively. Hans Baba joined their ranks at the Vindhyachal *ashram*, the place itself reverberating with spiritual charge.

Vindhyachal

Vindhyachal, a sleepy suburb near Varanasi, with thick forests and the world's oldest mountain range of the Vindhyas landscaping it, also happens to be a *Shaktipitha* and abode of *Vindhyavasini Devi.* Ancient sages are believed to have meditated in the Vindhya forests for thousands of years suffusing them with the powers of their own. Goddess *Vindhyavasini* is believed to fulfil the just wishes of scores of supplicants who visit the hills. The *ashram* itself is some 10 kms. away from the Vindhyachal temple.

A word about the wish fulfilling Goddess Vindhyavasini, whose story dates back to the times of Krishna's legendary birth. Kansa, the evil ruler of Mathura and Krishna's own maternal uncle, killed one by one, seven newborns of sister Devaki in the prisons. The killings stemmed from fearing a divine prophecy that the evil king was destined to be destroyed by Devaki's eighth child. At midnight on the *ashtami* day, was then born boy Krishna, only to be divinely whisked away to the safety of cowherd Nanda's house across a flooded Yamuna. Father Vasudeva who carried Krishna to Nanda's house was then to carry Nanda's new born daughter back to the prisons for hoodwinking Kansa who had reason to fear only a male offspring of Devaki. Yet, Kansa took no chances and resolved to slay the new-born female. As he drew out his sword and aimed it at the child, she magically flew off to the skies and solemnly made this prophecy on her way to the heavens, "Kansa, beware! Your killer has already been born!" That divine girl was *Yogamaya,* the

Goddess, and since she took it upon her to stay in the Vindhya hills ever since, she was called the *Vindhyavasini.* It appears to be of no mean spiritual significance in these troubled times, that the same legendary Vindhya hills were first inhabited by the great Devraha Baba and are now coming alive with the divine presence of Hans Baba.

Hans Becomes Paramahans

Even as the great fire of illumination was consuming Hans in the long and unsung years of *Sadhana* at the Vindhyachal *ashram*, his Guru was quietly preparing to permanently leave, first the *ashram* and then the mortal frame itself. Hans, the Guru knew, had arrived to keep going the *Siddha* tradition. Old timers recall that when some devotees approached an elusive Devraha Baba at Vrindavana and requested him to come back to the Vindhyachal *ashram*, the Guru advised them instead to go to Hans, who 'had become a Siddha'. It was not long thereafter that Devraha Baba cast away his mortal frame by calmly entering the Yamuna waters at Vrindavana, leaving Hans and lacks of devotees, crestfallen. He rushed to Vrindavana and then set off for the Himalayas in search of his departed Guru, who he knew, survived the physical body. Deep in the Himalayas, Hans ventured close to Gyanganj, a sacred zone believed to be inhabited only by men of God in their astral forms. Hans, once again bent upon giving up his physical frame by audaciously trying to enter the snowy Gyanganj territories against all climatic odds, was this time saved by the Guru who first appeared as a disembodied Voice and then, when Hans insisted, in his recognizable physical form. Following the Guru's command, Hans came back to the Vindhyachal *ashram* and, in a fit of inspiration, ascended the 'throne'. In one stroke, the *Bharata* was become Rama, and this news spread like wild fire throughout eastern and northern India. The news itself evoked a mixed reaction among the bereaved followers of Devraha Baba. Over the years, most of the original followers of the departed yogi have accepted Hans as an incarnate of the great Guru, though others continue to have reservations. Hans himself, his manners and bearings become strikingly like Devraha Baba's, began saying matter–of-factly that 'he was indeed Devraha Baba' and that 'Hans had flown away'. Could then Hans be a reincarnate of Devraha Baba? And if so, in what way, specially as the two *Siddhas* were both physically alive and together for several years?

Instances of a *Siddha* Guru keeping the tradition alive by transferring his spiritual power to his *Siddha* disciple shortly before his physical end, abound in the Yoga tradition. Ramakrishna did this with Vivekananda and wept that he was 'now left a beggar'. More recently, Guru Nityananda and Swami Muktananda formed such an illustrious pair. In the case of Devraha Baba and his *Siddha* disciple Hans however, things become a bit more complex as what is involved is transfer of the Guru's very being, rather than of his powers, to the worthy disciple. Yet, if we recall, too much should not be read into the apparently 'solid' and 'material' nature of our physical body that after all is nothing but an illusion. In the ultimate analysis, our physical body is a body made of 'nothing', conjured up by vibrating thoughts, ideas and impressions that occur in the stream of consciousness. In the transcendental world of a *Siddha* therefore, his physical, astral and purely spiritual forms are ever trans-mutating realities capable of manifesting as matter, thought or energy at his slightest command. In any case, *parakaya pravesha* or the ability of the soul to leave one physical body at will and enter another, is one of the *Siddhis* that, according to the yoga theory, accrues to the *Siddhas*. The great Shaivite yogi of the medieval times, Sankaracharya is believed to have used this ability to good effect in the cause of the Vedanta. (According to the *Shiva—Samhita* the yogin who awakens the third of the seven *chakras*—the *manipura*—gains the ability to leave his body and enter another. For a *Siddha*, who has gone far beyond and awakened all seven *chakras*, this should really be child's play!)

These polemics however, are barren and better avoided. As K. N. Rao has so succinctly put it, Hans Baba is an illumined yogi in his own right and this alone should matter to his devotees. To those of us who have seen the glory of this living saint, his lineage and psycho-physical linkages with Devraha Baba's erased physical entity are not of any great concern. Many disciples who were spiritually initiated by Devraha Baba 20 or 30 years back continue to see their master in Hans Baba. On the other hand, many seekers of the relatively younger generation, me included, have had no glimpse of Hans Baba's legendary Guru, and yet are none the poorer for it, having received the Grace of this living saint.

Looking Back

The first impression of Hans Baba is that of an ascetic, as if an ancient Himalayan sage had mistakenly strayed into our times and territories to give us, if nothing else, then a cultural shock. Seated on a raised wooden platform or a *machan*, he appears to be totally unmindful of the needs of his body. When I first saw him at Patna in the winters of 1997, his *machan* was just next to the Ganga with no brick structure screening the holy man from the icy winds that were blowing across the Ganga waters. In that extreme cold, we shivered and shrunk inside layers of warm clothing—pullovers, overcoats and all. And he sat majestically, clad in just a scanty loin cloth, with least concern for the near freezing cold in the wee hours of the morning or at the dead of night. To the discerning, seeing him like that was partly believing what the scriptures mean when they say that a *Siddha* has complete control over nature and his self. Since then, I have keenly observed him many times at Vindhyachal and Delhi, during the scorching Indian summer of May/June and also in the thundering monsoons of July/August. Each time I have found him unruffled, unconcerned with nature's fury, worrying instead all the time about the comfort of the visitors. In these difficult times, to me he appears as a man with a mission, even as a man in a hurry. 'Operating' from his base in Vindhyachal, he travels, mostly by road, extensively and tirelessly, to bless more and more lands and people across more and more townships. Once arrived at the destination, all he needs to seat himself and bless the thronging crowds therefrom, is another of those *machans* in a relatively open space. The logistics, including the *prasada* that he distributes, is generally provided by the willing and the capable among the local disciples. His whole body glistens; his disarming smile, his radiating eye contacts, his utterances all create a quaint old world charm more befitting of those ancient *Vedic* times.

Unlike his Guru, the departed Devraha Baba who was at least 200 years old when he took *Samadhi*, Yogi Hans Baba is a recent phenomenon. He came into reckoning and gained prominence, only after Devraha Baba left his mortal frame in 1990. But such is the magnificence of this yogi that within a decade of emergence and without any publicity whatsoever, Hans Baba has come to be venerated as a prophet-saviour by lakhs of people in eastern and northern India. I have never had the privilege of meeting Devraha Baba, so I cannot really compare these two spiritual giants. But some how, Hans Baba reminds me so much of the great Ramakrishna whose life and ways have been vividly portrayed among others, by Romain Rolland and Christopher Isherwood. The same disarming manners! The same radiant smile! The same piercing glances! The same lack of concern with bodily comforts and scholastic learning! The same bewildering tales of frolicking with Gods and Goddesses (there with Kali and Rama, here with Radha and Krishna!), the same lotus like aloofness amidst maddening crowds!

Trying to fully understand or describe a *Siddha* like Hans Baba is a hopeless task. What I have attempted instead, is a brief introduction. Summing up, I would like my reader to recall these words of Yogananda –

"Invariable rules may not be formulated about God – illumined saints; some perform miracles; others do not; some are inactive, while others......... are concerned with large affairs; some teach, travel and accept disciples, while others pass their lives as silently and unobtrusively as a shadow. No worldly critic can read the secret scroll of karma that unrolls for each saint a different script."

(Paramahansa Yogananda, *Autobiography of a Yogi*. Los Angeles: Self-Realization Fellowship, 1998)

To Recap

1. *Siddhas* or the God-realized saints are the rarest of rare beings, chances of finding whom is further diminished by their normally inaccessible ways.
2. Fortunately, some *Siddhas*, perhaps with a Divine Design, still roam among the masses blessing more and more people without compromising on the purity of the *Siddha* lineage.
3. One such *Siddha* is Yogi Hans Baba who is the worthy disciple of the great Devraha Baba and is believed by many to be his incarnate through the yogic technique of *para-kaya pravesha.*
4. Hans Baba is based at his *ashram* at Vindhyachal, the place having added sanctity by way of it being the abode of Goddess Vindhya-vasini.
5. Like all *Siddhas*, Hans Baba is loathe to parading his supernormal powers, but miracles keep happening around him specially in the form of miracle–cures that are legion.
6. In the delightfully inscrutable ways of the God-play, nothing happens per chance; when time is ripe, the Guru finds the disciple, rather than the other way round.

X. Healing the Future

"When the electron vibrates, the universe shakes."
—Sir Arthur Eddington

Healing the Future?

Healing the future! From the outset, I was clear about this being the title of the book. For, I wanted to emphatically convey that the process of healing that yoga triggers, is much deeper than anything that the physical scientists or even the average yoga expert could imagine. "What cannot be cured, must be endured", is the popular saying, and yoga's ability to increase man's endurance in face of adversity, is now too well documented and publicized to need any elaboration. Not many yoga practitioners however, get to know the equally big secret of yoga-practice, viz., its capacity *to cure what cannot be endured.* I have strived, however inadequately, to cover this extremely complex and controversial aspect of yoga in the chapter, *Planets and Free Will.* Carrying on from there, I would begin by describing the Hindu concept of disease from which the understanding of health automatically follows. As we have seen in the preceding chapters, the human form is supposed to comprise not one but many *bodies*—the gross one of our everyday perception and then the subtle bodies that are arranged in a descending order of coarseness. We have also seen how modern science is now beginning to unveil the first signs of these subtle bodies through means such as kirlian photography. The Ayurveda says that any disease first strikes the subtle bodies and only in due course manifests itself in the physical form. But what gives rise to the disease in the etheric planes in the first place? Here we have to go back to the theory of Karma that holds the key to the Hindu Thought that has fathered yoga. While at this stage we need not go into the nitty-gritty of the Karma principle, we can ill-afford to deal with the process of health and disease bereft of this background. According to the 'law of karma', *all human diseases are the direct consequence of one's accumulated bad karmas of present and past lives, with the cosmic objective of creating within the subject such suffering as to push him towards introspection and some serious soul-searching assuming that in the mad hedonistic pursuit, it was never attempted before.* Edward Bach, British physician, writing in "*Heal Thyself : An Explanation of the Real Cause and Cure of Disease*" held that disease was essentially beneficial, with the design to subject the individual to Divine Will. Clearly then, any recipe for good health or freedom from disease has to be not only three-dimensional, but a transcendental one.

The real import of the above thesis however, is this. Let us return to the position that past negative karmas of this life and before result in physical disease. Is that all? The answer is a resounding "No". Scriptures leave us in no doubt that our past karmas not only give rise to our physical state of ease and disease, but they also shape each and every twist of our future: the fears, the insecurities, the hopes, the aspirations, the failures, the successes, career, finances, and so on. It follows therefore that a prescription for *healing*, in the widest sense of the term, would be one that attempts to neutralize the very currents of one's past negative karmas through 'an equal and opposite force' that would have a curative influence not only on his physical health, but on his entire future, penetrating all aspects of life, mundane and spiritual. Hence the title of this chapter. I have arranged the suggested moves towards a healthier and more fulfilling life in the English alphabetical arrangement in an attempt to consciously and subconsciously convince the reader that, while the goal may be distant, initiating the process of 'future-healing' and gaining rich dividends therefrom is as elementary and interesting as the nursery rhyme.

The Alphabet of Healing

I do not have to go into the theory behind the yoga process all over again, which has been amply covered in the preceding chapters. The present chapter is exclusively about its utilitarian face, intended to provide the reader with the most practical tips that may look deceptively simple, yet go a long way in setting off the process of healing that culminates in Yoga. As mentioned earlier, I have taken utmost care to ensure authenticity of all information and narratives contained in this book which, let me assure you, was not an easy task given their abstract character. The authenticity factor however, becomes paramountly significant in this particular chapter since it is all about practice, not precept of yoga and has a direct bearing on the reader's physical and mental well-being. In this sense, the present chapter is more like the doctor's prescription, than like the theologist's benign discourses. With this important difference however, that healing envisaged here is not limited in its objective to curing physical diseases, but is geared to bring about a complete three-dimensional overhauling that attempts nothing less than putting your destiny, in large measures, in your own hands. Truely, it does not merely promise to *take darkness out of the night*; it makes you try to greatly *hasten the sunrise itself*. If I am beginning to sound guilty of the same populism and short-cut that I have earlier cautioned the reader against, consider these important differences. Unlike the many pseudo-techniques of the New Age, the prescriptions given here do not cost the earth. Nor do they ask you to visit this or that centre in what may turn out to be a camouflage for money–minting and cult-promotion. What is suggested instead is a regimen of 'do it yourself' exercises—

in simple, easy-to-master steps. Most of the practical tips that find mention here are either born of my own experience, or culled from authentic sources of the great *Siddha* tradition of the East. On many occasions I have also tried to seamlessly weld my own perceptions with the wisdom received from the scriptures, genuine scholars and my own *Siddha* Guru. For example, when I prescribe *japa* with the aid of a conscious mantra as a holistic remedy for your depression and diseases, I am speaking very much from my own valuable experience. On the other hand, when I dwell on the same *japa* as possible means to changing the currents of your destiny, I am relying largely on the observations of my Guru, views of great astrologers like K. N. Rao and the legacy of seers of the recent past. Even in seemingly as innocuous a thing as water therapy, I have prescribed simple chores which I learnt through authentic texts and /or practised back home with ample rewards. Before I come to the *alphabet of healing* let me also clarify once again that it is a language which I am myself learning all the time and which I want to share with my readers by becoming one of them rather than by standing on an ivory tower.

The phonetic inadequacy of the English language and *'the unsuccessful struggle of 26 English letters to bear the burden of sound'* are too well known to be repeated. Considering however, that English continues to be the most accepted language internationally, I now propose to make use of the same 26 alphabets in a novel way, viz., by making them 'bear the burden of healing'. So here we go:

A — Astrological Counsel
B — Bhagavad Gita
C — Charity
D — Diet
E — Egoctomy
F — Fasting
G — Guru
H — Humours

I — Introspection
J — *Japa*
K — Karma concept
L — Laughter
M — Music
N — Nature care
O — *Ojas*
P — Physical *asana*
Q — Questioning
R — Regularity
S — Slowing down
T — Travelling
U — Uncork
V — Vegetarianism
W — Water therapy
X — X-Zone
Y — *Yoga-nidra*
Z — Zeroing in

A. Astrological Counsel

The subject has been discussed threadbare in the chapter *'Planets and Free Will'*. To make full use of your inherent yoga potential, try to become more self–aware in the first place. Even if you are suffering from mild depression or are unable to handle stress, a single visit to an insightful astrologer may successfully replace hundreds of time–and–money consuming sessions with psychiatrists and clinical psychologists, unless of course, you are (hopefully correctly) diagnosed with a medical condition that necessitates intake of drugs. In which case the astrologer's counselling may still be a nice supplement to the doctor's prescription.

If you have reasonably accurate details of the date, time and place of your birth—which in all likelihood you do by way of the hospital certificate or in the family tradition—make brisk use of technology. Get your birth horoscope cast by a computer in ten minutes flat; make sure that you go for the economy version that contains only the calculations and not the actual forecasts that are best left in the cares of a good astrologer with his intuitive insight. This would save your astrologer days of manual labour and enable him to straightaway come to the analysis part. Don't be fearful or superstitious; good astrologers are good psychologists as well. They will encourage you to follow profitable leads while detailing the goodness contained in your birth chart with hints on how to maximize it, and generally couch the unpleasant forebodings in soft language, to be discerned and be guarded against by the astute among the consultors. Remember always that you have come to see the astrologer not to know an 'unalterable future' (such a thing does not exist) but to be enlightened about *future probabilities* whose *pluses* can then be exploited and *minuses*, muted through Yoga.

To cite my own example, in view of my badly afflicted Sun in the natal chart, I was cautioned against a possible heart attack during my Sun major period in very early 50s. A daily recital of the *Aditya Hrdaya Stotra* (a Sanskrit hymn to Sun God culled from the *Valmiki Ramayana*) might help—it was gingerly suggested. Part-scared, part-stung, I tried reciting the hymn only to find the pronunciation so difficult as to be nearly given up. *"No,"* came the assurance, *"your charts indicate that you will not only do successful Sadhana through hymns and mantra, but also go deeper and deeper in meditation"*. Encouraged, yet full of doubts, I once again gave it a try, and viola! I mastered the pronunciation and remembered the entire hymn with effortless ease within two days—so much so that it appeared to be a small miracle in its own right. The *Aditya Hrdaya Stotra*, true to its promise, took me deep into meditation and, at least I believe it that way, exposed me to circumstances and scriptural readings that were divinely designed to usher me into Shaktipat-yoga. *"Sir, does my horoscope indicate diksha"*, I tentatively put this question to K. N. Rao during my first meeting with him at his Delhi residence in the middle of 1997. *"Yes, but a little later*", came the assurance. "*And does my horoscope indicate a stroke during the Sun major period?*", I grew more inquisitive. "*No, all this will be taken care of by the japa. A sadhaka should not worry about the future once he takes diksha,*" was the reply from a stern looking Rao. Implicit here was perhaps this great astrologer's knowledge that for a genuinely initiated *sadhaka* sincerely practising *japa*, the vice-like grip of planets begins to loosen making his future more 'unpredictable' than the run-of-the-mill astrologers and laymen would imagine. Sure enough, I got spiritually initiated by Hans Baba sooner than later at his Vindhyachal *ashram*, after a six month long hide and seek game with the omniscient Guru, who inevitably prevailed without talking much. To this day, I marvel how a completely lazy and sceptical person like me, gravitated towards deeper and deeper modes of yoga almost *in spite of oneself*. 'Destiny and Guru's Grace', is the ready answer, but astrology played its part as well, first putting the fear of God in me, and then showing the way out. What if prediction of an imminent heart attack early on, had shattered me and brought the 'inevitable' even closer in time? It is here that choice of the astrologer and your own sense of proportions, become crucial. Like when you choose your Guru, the astrologer to be sought must be a low profile man, preferably a non-professional, whose reputation as a good astrologer was authentic enough to justify a visit. The astrologer who brags too much, declares that he can make or mar your destiny, has an air of finality about his forecasts, and directly or indirectly peddles gems, talismans and *yantras*, is best avoided.

The good astrologer would rather prescribe a hymn or a mantra for propitiation of planets, such as the *Aditya Hrdaya* for Sun, the *Hanuman Chalisa* for Saturn and Mars, and the *Rama Raksha Stotra* or simply the *Gayatri mantra* for all purposes. Charity and fasting on a particular day may also be prescribed. Wearing of gems is also recommended, but this is an area mired in controversy. To start with, this is a very expensive affair with most precious gems costing tens of thousand of rupees in India. Secondly there is no guarantee of the genuineness of the stone regardless of what the seller tells you. Thirdly and most importantly, different astrologers, even if they broadly agree on the readings of your horoscope, differ markedly in prescribing gems. If however, you happen to be cash-rich and also in touch with a really good astrologer who knows gems inside out, I personally believe that gems do have a place in yoga and should be made use of after due consideration.

Those who are already initiated by a *Siddha* Guru, may not need either the hymns or the gems, since *the conscious mantra is the highest vehicle of Yoga.* Those who are not yet *Shaktipat-initiated,* and also find the Sanskrit hymns difficult to pronounce, specially the Westerners, need not despair. For them, a loving and faithful recital of the seed mantra 'Om' (Aum) on a daily basis can have the same effect as that of the hymns. In the end, there is a small piece of advice that I believe, does work and obviates the need for astrological prognostication owing to its universal efficacy. Wear a *rudraksha mala* of 108 beads. The beads, that are best got from *Rishikesha,* should be genuine and small enough for convenience, and the *mala* should be worn at all times, except during sex.

B. Bhagavad Gita

The Bhagavad Gita needs no introduction to the billions of Easterners across the world, or even to the yoga conscious West. Today, in the average Hindu household, this ancient treatise on Hindu spiritualism takes the pride of place at the worship place. However, one very much doubts if even one per cent of the Hindu intelligentsia, not to talk of the rest, takes the pain to actually read it from beginning to end even once, save in the twilight of their lives. If however, you venture forth, you will find that, quite aside from its ecclesiasticism, it has the most insightful yogic lessons for the secular minded. Approached from the point of view of the Gita, meditation is no more or less Hindu than sleep is Muslim or dreams are Christian. That the Gita expounds the universally applicable principle of detached action and goes on to most insightfully "reveal" the great treasure of kriya-yoga, pranayama together with esoteric mind–management techniques, is now being increasingly acknowledged world-wide. A dispassionate reading of the *Gita* purely as a Yoga scripture is likely to unravel the hidden divine messages in the *Qoran*, and the *Old and New Testaments* to the non-Hindu yoga aspirants.

The popular misconception that Gita's karma-yoga dispenses the psychologically impracticable advice of *doing one's work while forgetting the goal,* has somehow lingered over the years. A serious first hand exposure to the original text, or one of its authentic English/Vernacular translations, would instead, go a long way in helping the yoga practitioner to become more focused and adept in his mundane pursuits by his not worrying too much about the possible consequences. Even modern psychology confirms that in relatively more complex situations, the efficiency curve when plotted against the arousal level, takes an inverted U shape. In other words, *too much arousal or eagerness to achieve the goal actually hinders goal accomplishment.* In high skill games, such as cricket and tennis, players are advised to 'take it easy' and not to try too much, lest the pressure of expectations gets to them.

C. Charity

In scriptures, along with penance and mantra, charity is prescribed as one of the chief means of lessening the rigours of life through planetary propitiation. The word charity in the yogic context however, means much more than is ordinarily implied. In yoga, just as matter, thought and energy are all fundamentally one, so is charity in thought or action, essentially identical. Charity does not therefore, exclusively lie in giving away precious material things in alms. *A noble thought directed at the other, a desire to share someone's suffering, a pat on your subordinate's back at the work place, a readiness to forgive and forget, are all examples of charity.* The Gita recognizes the concept of unmanifest karma that refers to actions that were thought of, but for some reason, fell short of execution. For example, if I am a young man courting a girl friend and catch her two-timing, I seethe with anger and feel like killing her. (Some would go ahead and do just that regardless!) But for the laws, the feared repercussions and a possible backlash of my own conscience, I would actually kill her. Eventually, outwardly I am seen to have 'done nothing'. In yoga theory however, I have already killed her in thought which is different only in degrees from killing her physically. Although an actual murder would definitely hold much more serious *karmic* consequences, the very desire to kill that lingered on and held me captive for long periods has become my negative karma. Now take the reverse for a proper understanding of charity. There is a little boy drowning in the river and ten people jump at a time to save him. Only one eventually comes anywhere near the child and saves him. You happen to be among the remaining nine who are left with nothing to do but feel relieved at the happy ending of the crisis. Although you and eight others have apparently done nothing to save the child, you have actually credited a lot of charity in your spiritual 'bank balance'.

Charity in order to be real charity, must have two other characteristics which *prima-facie* look rooted in nature (as if you can do nothing consciously about it) but which can be gradually cultivated to become part of your personality. These are: *(a) an element of sacrifice, and (b) a degree of selflessness.* In the same example, if out of the ten people, nine others were good swimmers secure in this knowledge, and you were the odd-man-out who did not know a thing about swimming and yet dived to save the child, risking your own life, your charity, in the *karmic* scheme of things; is the greatest, possibly even outweighing the charity of the lone swimmer who actually saved the child. (Implicit here is *Gita's* concept of our being the *medium* rather than the *source* of all phenomena.) A final word about selflessness or the ability to lie low after doing charity. Of the ten good Samaritans, if nine others went back to the town, trumpeting their bravery, and if the lone successful rescuer also secretly expected the child's parents to suitably reward him, charity has ceased to be thus any longer. It has degenerated into barter and their 'savings accounts' show little credit. On the other hand, you hear of the incident back in your office and read about it in the newspapers, yet do not let it be known that you were one of the famous ten. Truly then, your act of charity has become *karmically* magnified many times over.

As a *karmic* remedy, charity can therefore, be effective only if *it flows from within, selflessly and silently.* The actual outcome of the intended charity—its shape and size—is largely incidental, divinely controlled and therefore of much lesser *karmic* consequence than commonsense would suggest. Agreed, charity going by the above description, is hard to achieve. Remember however, that it is all a matter of degrees and fusion. As you practise bit by bit this language of yoga, each of the alphabets has unknown to you, forged, individually and holistically, living ties with each of the twenty-five other types of yoga. Charity that started artificially as a self-seeking astrological remedy, may soon be impacted by the truth learnt from Gita, a vegetarian diet, fasting, introspection and *japa* and sundry other practices to become a living reality that thrives on its own. As for me, honestly, I am these days trying to consciously avoid making 'uncharitable' remarks against colleagues and relatives who tend to be difficult. And believe me, it has not been as easy as it sounds! The big lesson of charity is best learnt in small steps, and not to think ill of anybody in trying circumstances can be just the kind of charity to get us started. In the end, be ware that *the law of karma is such that each negative or positive thought directed at others is, in effect a boomerang!*

D. Diet

There is no exaggeration in the saying that *we are what we eat.* K. N. Rao goes so far as to say that *80 percent of Sadhana is right diet.* The yoga practitioner has to be particular about his eating, since even on a day-to-day basis, diet has a strong influence on the physical and astral bodies. It is nobody's case that food should not be tasteful. However, the practice of yoga over a period of time, brings about subtle changes in the palate and the taste buds themselves whereby you would be naturally drawn to the right food and drinks. Hot spices, salt, coffee and meat are foods that agitate the mind and interfere with yoga. Most of us eat 10 to 20 times more salt than recommended, the recommended daily intake being only 6 grams or one tea-spoonful. Most of this salt comes indirectly through canned food/restaurant meals etc.—something best avoided on most occasions. A high salt intake increases the risk of high blood pressure, osteoporosis ,cardiovascular disease and kidney troubles. Nearly half of the adult US population is at the high blood pressure threshold or above, and to make things worse, blood pressure normally increases with age. Bottom line: less salt means more health.

As to the intake of onions and garlic, there is some debate on this issue in that while the puritans reject it altogether as *rajasika* or negative, they are of obvious nutritional value to the physical body. Personally, I would advise the reader to take the utilitarian middle path—cut down intake of raw onions and garlic to nourish your astral bodies without denying your physical body an occasional helping. The early morning intake of raw garlic–cloves can be easily replaced with one tablespoonful of dried *methi* (fenugreek) + *amla* (Indian gooseberry) powder, with equally impressive medicinal and nutritive results. (The extreme step of completely avoiding onions-and–garlic based cooking in your kitchen, unless you are used to it beforehand, is better avoided at least at the initial stages.) Similarly, all canned and processed food should be gradually given up, as also the habit of smoking. Sugar-intake should be cut down and substituted, wherever possible, with honey and jaggery. (*Just one spoonful of sugar cuts the response of infection fighting white blood cells by half, and this effect lasts for a full five hours*!) Giving up alcohol seems to be a lot more difficult and in any case, contrary to the popular notion, alcohol and the wine specially, is much less damaging than meat-eating and smoking. If you enjoy an occasional peg in the right circles, you do not have to despair. With the yoga practice, all of these addictions are bound to gradually fall away on their own owing to the subtle changes that occur in the nervous system and in the levels of consciousness. Fresh fruits, vegetables, sprouts, yogurt and honey must start contributing much more to your daily intake. For, a subtle portion of the diet becomes your consciousness and its grossness is gradually removed with a healthier diet, greatly helping the yoga process.

E. Egoctomy

The *Siddhas* never tire of telling you to 'empty yourself' for the divine consciousness to enter and illuminate your inner spaces. Scriptures clearly say that *all human actions result from a combination of the three ever-active 'gunas'—tamasika* (the sloth principle), *rajasika* (the activity principle) *and sattvika* (the brightness principle)—and that *man in his vanity, thinks of himself as the doer*. The dominant feeling of *ahamkara* or I-ness results in big talking, hurting others, inaccurate reality perception and a host of other undesirable behavioural patterns that in any case, reduce your social acceptability and cause relational conflicts. The person who talks less of himself and makes others feel important is invariably the more liked in a group. To think of yourself as nothing is however, not the same as harbouring an inferiority complex. As you consciously go about emptying yourself, the yoga process will impact you with ever quickening impulses to make you happy, centred and confident. A good way to start is by gratefully telling yourself and others of how others bailed you out in times of need, rather than how you helped them. And when the ego still gets big on you, just pause and remember the lessons learnt from physics—you are, in the most literal sense, '*nothing*'.

F. Fasting

In yoga, fasting is advised for physical healing as well as for spiritual implications. Doctors, specially in the West are divided in their opinion as to the actual effects of rigorous fasting on the body. Some nutrition experts are in fact of the opinion that fasting is actually counterproductive. The theory that sees fasting as a healing process however, still holds its ground based on its own logic: *during a long fasting, the detoxification process sets in. The sugar reserves in the liver and muscles are burnt up. The body attempting to conserve energy, goes easy on many vital organic functions, which in turn aids tissue-repair and recuperation. The energy otherwise required for digestion, now accelerates immune activity, cell growth and expulsion of waste. With the stored sugar used up, the body starts burning fat reserves to meet the energy requirement. Toxins, heavy metals and pesticides deposited in the fat tissues through years of indiscreet eating and drinking are, in the process thrown out. Fasting also leads to a thinner blood that improves circulation of oxygen and white blood cells in the entire system.*

Stomach complains, kidney troubles, arthritis, headache and heart diseases are some of the major conditions in which fasting has been seen to help. However those suffering from cancer, ulcers, tuberculosis and thyroid disorders should generally avoid fasting. In any case, fasting must be undertaken after due consultations with your physicians and a precautionary medical check up. Personally I would suggest that instead of going overboard, you resort to juice fasting i.e., take only fruit juices with helpings of curd and honey, avoiding cereals and salt. Benefits of fasting can become synergistic and yogic when it is attuned with astrological considerations. The seven days of the week correspond to nine planets, and fasting on a particular day propitiates a particular planet. Choose a fixed day for fasting every week after due astrological consultation.

G. Guru

Why to choose a Guru, how to choose and whom, has been amply covered under a previous chapter. Given the central role of Guru in unfolding of Yoga within, I would here reiterate the basic considerations. Choose a Guru who: *(a) does not care for money and publicity, (b) says what he does, (c) knows and disseminates the teachings of* scriptures, *(d) does not talk too much and (e) makes you feel at peace in his presence.* Beyond these elementary precautions however, getting a *Siddha* Guru is a matter of *destiny* rather than *choice*. Do not therefore loose your sleep over how and where to find the Guru. When the time is ripe and the tidings come, the Guru 'chooses' you and not you, him. If any convincing on this point is required, then think of the example of Dr. B. Nayak in the chapter, *Yogi Hans Baba.*

H. Humours

The Ayurveda recognizes the presence of an internal equilibrium of three humours *(doshas)* or the lack of it as the basic causative factor in health or disease, (a) *vata*, or wind (b) *pittta,* or bile, and (c) *kapha* or phlegm. The three humours are essentially metabolic types. Each of the human beings is a unique blend of all the three types with one type generally dominant and largely determining our personality. Since Ayurveda is literally, the *science of life* and not of *disease*, each of us, in our attempt to become more self-aware, must be proactive and become conversant with our own humour type, regardless of our simplistic labels of *healthy* and *diseased.* Once you know your humour type, the necessary corrections in diet and life-style can be made in easy, small steps for removing the humour defects (*tridoshas*). Try to see a genuine Ayurvedic physician at least once, at the earliest. Let him feel your pulse (yes, this is the way an expert Ayurvedic physician gets to know your humour defect) and tell you your basic humour type. Whether you put yourself in his therapeutic care thereafter, is something that would depend on the diagnosis made and your own inclination. But the very awareness of your basic humour type and humour defect is a definite step forward in healing. To start with, you can also tentatively judge your humour by introspecting. Here are some useful hints:

(a) *vata*—energetic, impulsive, imaginative, anxious, insomniac, lean, having dry skin, prone to nervous disorders.
(b) *pitta*—efficient, punctual, perfectionist, intelligent, articulate, temperamental, of medium built, perspiring skin, prone to stomach disorders.
(c) *kapha*—relaxed, balanced, tolerant, procrastinating, obese, prone to allergy and high cholesterol problems.

I. Introspection

Closely allied with the idea of ego-surrendering is that of introspection. We have seen how the inner universe is virtually a replica of the vast outer universe. The great *rishis* of the past had neither the sophisticated tools nor the external means to discover the truths lying behind the bewildering range of phenomena. If they were yet able to acquire a degree of self-awareness and knowledge of the universe that is out of bounds for the most brilliant of modern physicists and consciousness researchers, it was made possible through introspection. For introspection in its concentrated form becomes intuition.

Since unravelling the mysteries of the universe is not likely to be of any immediate concern to most of us, we can be well served with relatively milder doses of introspection. Introspect however you must. For you do not realize your little follies and foibles unless you look inward. The Buddhist form of meditation that has been found so powerfully cleansing and vivifying for many of us, *Vipassana*, literally means 'looking inwards'. Constant introspection, when it becomes a habit, will rid your mind–body monolith of many oddities and complexes. It will also then enable you to creatively, subconsciously—even psychically—find solutions to knotty problems, thus raising your success–rate and self-esteem.

J. Japa

This again has been discussed at length earlier. *Japa* of the conscious mantra is the simplest and yet the most powerful of all yogic practices. It is unencumbered by constraints of time, money, intellect and rituals. Do the *japa* meditation determinedly at the beginning—starting with ten minutes and gradually increasing the duration to half an hour or more at a time. The key to successful *japa* is to *internally visualize the mantra and to feel it as pulsating and moving in every nook and corner of your head. The mantra must be repeated internally and as far as possible, without any movement of the lips, the tongue and the vocal cord. Your eyes should be closed, attention fixed at the third eye centre between the two eyebrows as far as possible, and the breath gradually made to chime with the mantra repetition. However, do not try too hard to either concentrate or synchronize the japa with breath. The mantra will have its own way and take its own rhythm in due course independent of your volition. Nor should you try to forcibly push out or screen the riot of apparently unconnected, meaningless, even offensive thoughts that initially bombard you as you sit meditating*. Be a silent *witness* rather than a *participant* or a *judge*, to the extent you can, and allow them to gradually fade away as you enter more peaceful states that come with practice. The beauty of the conscious *mantra* is that it is usually a very short one that can and should be repeated wherever and whenever the slightest opportunity presents itself. You must repeat it while eating, having your cup of tea, during travel, as you drive to the office, when taking bath, in your evening walk. *Japa*, as it becomes first a habit and then a beautiful addiction, is a most powerful cleanser that burns off your past negative karmas and impressions very fast giving you a new destiny.

K. Karma Concept

Often have I found, very intelligent people smugly excusing themselves out of yoga on the facile plea that they are already doing the needful by taking morning walks or going swimming, or doing aerobics. If anything, this makes me feel sorry for them, specially if I additionally, sense a tone of finality in their statement as if to shut the doors on any further discussion on the subject. For, what they are saying in effect, if I go back to the example I started with in this book, is that *'they don't have any use for the PC because they already have got one nice typewriter back home'*. No doubt daily morning walks and swimming are good physical exercises that have some refreshing effect on the nerves as well. But in their reach, balance and power to do good, the key yoga practices such as meditation compare with the purely physical exercises as an aircraft would, with a sports car . And if you also happen to be blessed by a *Siddha* Guru in the form of a live mantra, you have doubtless, upgraded the aircraft into a rocket. This rather picturesque comparison would explain itself once I add a few words on the crucially important concept of karma in this context—a concept much talked about, and yet, least understood.

The scriptures teach us about the different modes of action or karmas. *Sanchita karma*, as the name implies, is the sum-total of actions of the past lying in store to fructify. *Prarabdha* is that part of our past karmas that has to unfold in this life. And *Kriyamana karma* is our actions taking place 'now and here', for their reaction to be felt later. It is by qualitatively improving our *kriyamana karma* that we can alleviate our sufferings and root out our physical diseases.

Like a good billiards player does with the red and yellow/white balls, you should aim measured shots to earn you the bigger (spiritual) points with such deftness that the side-impacting automatically wins you the lesser (physical, mental) points. Remember once again that health is much more than physical well being, and that yoga–practice, unlike simple physical exercises, is intended for deliverance from *karmic* sufferings of all hues that go far beyond physical illness. Remember also, that if you are a diabetic, a heart patient, or carry a tumour, then it would be naive for you to expect yourself to 'walk', 'run' or 'swim' your way totally out of the *karmic* trap. If you have to escape misery wrought on the ground by *karmic* grooves of your own making, then you would have to eschew riding on the surface and take on the aerial route. The simple truth is that *concentrated yoga–practices such as meditation, powerfully act on the source viz., your karmic burdens, whereas isolated physical exercises cannot penetrate the surface.* So, next time you go out for a walk or a swimming session, enjoy yourself, but not at the expense of yoga.

L. Laughter

Along with the sensation of touch, laughter has remained at the centre of recent research to assess the therapeutic effects of the more natural among human responses. Strengthening of the immune system, a marked rise in energy levels, release of blockages and fixations, and improved functioning of the glandular and circulatory systems are some of the positive effects now well documented as resulting from bouts of hearty laughter. *In one study, 10 healthy people watched a funny video for an hour, and were then found to have significantly increased levels of gamma interferon, a cytokine hormone that activates key constituents of the immune system* . Our stiff upper-lipped society with all its sophistication and sham convictions, now puts a premium on laughing innocently and uninhibitedly. Instead, you are expected to be socially correct by allowing yourself just that wry smile. Feel free however, to laugh aloud and awhile each day in your privacy and amongst your more informal circles, if you want to live life. Occasions for such laughter will present themselves (remember what science has to say about perception—it is as much your own creation as registering of sensory input) once you mentally tune yourself to it. Meanwhile, privacy and informal relationships need assiduous cultivation for the right feel of yoga.

M. Music

We have already seen how rise of the entire universe is ultimately traced to sound, and how, carefully orchestrated sound in the 'shape' of mantras can be so powerfully yogic as to lead us to divinity. The other sound pattern that is much less esoteric, and yet having a like healing effect comes in the form of music. Music, the proverbial 'medicine of the mind' is primarily entertainment–stuff. True music however, *edifies* even as it *entertains*. Scientific studies documenting the ability of music to stimulate plant growth and enhance cattle yield are now legion. Although the salutary effect of music on man, with his much more complex nervous system and higher faculties is likely to be less straightforward, evidence emerging by the day of its high therapeutic value has triggered a whole new area of clinical practice in music therapy. Clinical researchers confirm that listening to music removes stress, lowers blood pressure and improves concentration. It also lessens nausea after chemotherapy, and greatly boosts creativity and motor-skills. *A study conducted at Yale University School of Medi-*

cine showed that people who listened to their preferred music while awake during surgery, needed relatively much smaller doses of sedatives and painkillers. The yoga theory recognizes music (*nada*) for what it is. In fact one way to characterize the seven *chakras* of the human astral body in the yoga system is to identify each *chakra* with one basic musical note, so as to symbolically grasp the entire human form together with the original musical *raga* or band of '*sa, re, ga, ma, pa, dha, ni, sa*'.

When you intend to tap into the therapeutic value of music, don't be too conscious of the therapeutic aspects. The current fads notwithstanding, the best music is always holistic; it entertains as much as it heals. The classical symphonies of Mozart, Beethoven and like masters of the West, as also the *Hindustani/Carnatic ragas* of the Indian tradition are all one in that they are yogic. If pure classical music appears to be a bit heavy, which I fear is often the case, I would strongly recommend light ghazals and the semi-classical (for the Hindi/Urdu knowing) music of the Hindi cinema of 1960s. It is pure bliss, embellished with captivating use of sounds from *Sitar,* the flute, the piano and like delicate instruments. Like mantras, this semi-classical music almost perfectly blends thought with sound. All fast and pop varieties of the latest music must however, be avoided. Studies as well as common sense suggest that this 'noise' that passes for music agitates the mind and interferes with yoga. Similarly the latest fashion of playing audio-cassettes and CDs of sacred Sanskrit *mantras* and hymns in the hope of some of it rubbing in, is a marketing gimmick in poor taste. *Mantras* in order to become effective must be *personally* and *internally* repeated, and are different from music in that they were never intended as entertainment. Like the seed of a Banyan tree in soil, *hymns and mantras need to be sown deep into the human consciousness, and tended with love and care, in order to grow and give shade.* Cassettes of *mantras* and hymns therefore, neither make true mantra nor good music. However recordings of '*bhajans*' or tasteful devotional songs are fine for company and for their soothing effect.

N. Nature Care

Take utmost care of your physical body, since it is a healthy body that paradoxically, would gradually enable you to rise above body consciousness that yoga demands. Unfortunately, in the Indian subcontinent and though less markedly, in the West as well, one of the prices that twentieth century man has had to pay for material progress, is loss of purity, both figuratively and literally. To talk here of the literal sense only, we breathe air that is foul, drink water that is contaminated and eat food that is adulterated. As if the daily mandatory doses of pesticides, chemical fertilizers, heavy metals, toxic automobile fumes and a host of other poisons were not good enough, there is this exponentially growing risk of nuclear contamination of atmospheric air and water in the high seas from radioactive releases. Disasters such as the recent sinking of the Russian nuclear submarine that killed the 150-odd crew and is now said to threaten the lives of millions with its precariously lying nuclear fissile matter in the deep seas, are feared to be ticking time bombs for humanity. (For some cosmic reason, these natural and man-made disasters are greatly on the rise of late. Reliable *Vedic* astrologers, specially K. N. Rao, foresee the period 1999 to 2002 as particularly difficult for humanity at large.)

While nothing much can be done individually by us to change the ways of the world so as to stop the sailing of a nuclear submarine in the high seas or even order all the damned automobiles off the road (except ours!), there is still a lot we can do. We are potentially, masters of our inner universe, which if you remember, is virtually a replica of the outer world impacting it significantly. How profoundly this inner universe influences the outer world, can be gauged from this remarkable observation of John W. Armstrong, author of *The Water of Life* that *those men who fomented or were responsible for wars were not healthy people—Julius Caeser was an epileptic, Napolean, a cancer-victim and Hitler, a neurasthenic of the worst kind.*

The most important step that therefore, we can take is to *return to Mother Nature* in the body's upkeep and repair. Increasingly, allopathy has been found wanting in giving us holistic and enduring solutions to our health problems notwithstanding the impressive advances made in surgical and diagnostic techniques. Allopathy is admittedly a necessity for the common man in times of emergency and in conditions requiring surgical intervention. There is also no denying that the recent breakthroughs in medicine and surgery have made the allopathic treatment a lot less invasive. Yet few among the thinking would contest that the end results of allopathic treatment are still far from encouraging, with diseases ranging from the dreaded cancer and AIDS, to the common cold showing no signs of capitulation. *Patients taking antibiotics have been found to carry reduced levels of cytokines, the hormone messengers of the immune system, as compared to others.* Some medical scientists have also begun doubting the efficacy of an increasing number of vaccines, even suspecting their possible roles in the markedly rising levels of heart and cancer diseases. If legally and psychologically allopathy still continues to have an iron hold on man's psyche and physique, it has a lot to do with extraneous considerations which however, cannot but be central to the billion-dollared pharmaceutical multinationals and the worldwide medical fraternity in this age of consumerism. John W. Armstrong, writing in '*The Water of Life*', incisively discerned *the curious irony in the fact that the treatment of certain allegedly incurable diseases had become illegal except at the hands of those who could not cure them! He likened this oddity to a law then existing in one of the American States that made it illegal for a husband to kiss his wife on a Sunday! With this important difference that unlike this particular piece of legislation, the equally strange law on medicine involved huge commercial interests: serums and radium plants, quite unlike a kiss, being manufacturable commodities.*

Among the methods that make use of nature in treatment, *Acupuncture* might make you uneasy with the fear of the needle in this age of AIDS and Hepatitis B. *Acupressure* however is fine, and sure to greatly benefit your condition irrespective of whether outwardly you suffer from an ailment or not. (Remember health and disease form a continuum and bodily disturbances, when they take roots, take a long time to surface as disease.) Take a break from your hectic routine this weekend, and get to know more of this ancient Chinese technique of manipulating your inner energies and 'meridians' by visiting the nearby expert. Aromatherapy that makes use of essential oil extracts from flowers, may also be in order for enhancing the yoga mood, although this may turn out to be more expensive. Recall that smell is the only sensory input to go directly to the brain, screened only by the hypothalamus. Homeopathy also holds much promise along with its much simpler version of *Biochemic* medicine that relies on twelve 'tissue' salts to replenish the deficient inorganic substances in the blood/tissues and thus destroy the breeding ground for the fungi, germs and bacilli. Today, a first-aid Homeopathic/Biochemic kit of ready-to-serve medicinal combinations catering to specific diseases such as diarrhoea, headache, flu, fever and flatulence is available off the shelf. And trust me, it is quite a help in times of need, once you know the basics. Though holistic, safe and potent, the chief drawback of Homeopathy lies in its dependence on correct diagnosis that many times eludes the obscure practitioner. A good homeopath once told me that depending on the particular patient, there are a possible 300 types of Homeopathic medicines or their combinations to treat one single disease of asthma! In *Bach Flower Therapy*, developed by Edward Bach in 1930s, the unique healing powers of 38 wild flowers are said to have been 'psychically' discovered by him, with the life force of each of these flowers being transferable to water and thence, to humans.

To me it appears nonetheless, that the Ayurveda holds the key to man's relative emancipation from disease and disorder in the New Age. Having its genesis in the Vedas, the Ayurveda is the most yogic of all medicinal techniques and has one suspects, finally 'arrived'. By using the latest mass manufacturing and processing techniques that were till recently the preserve of the medical orthodoxy, reputed Indian Ayurvedic companies have combined the benefits of the new and the old schools synergistically. Feel free to use the diagnostic and surgical methods of Allopathy in times of real need. Trust however, a clever mix of the right food and right natural medicine to aid the body's innate intelligence in enabling you to remain fighting fit.

O. Ojas

Celibacy is an alien concept to the Western culture which is marked by permissiveness and indiscriminate indulgence. A strictly celibate life is neither possible nor necessary for yoga practitioners at large. Yet, the yoga tradition is emphatic that *creative energy is dissipated in sexual experience, and conserved in celibacy*. The Cosmic life force or *prana*, sustains and moves the outer universe in its external aspect, while it manifests on the physical level as sexual energy in its internal aspect. The sexual energy normally moves in the downward direction and gets used up in sex act. However, *if a degree of sexual economy is observed along with other key yoga practices such as meditation and diet discipline, the same sexual energy begins to flow upwards in the form of ojas*. Ojas is the quintessential nourishing essence that is to be found in the bone-marrows and is distributed over the entire body. However, the greatest concentration of *ojas* is in semen (*bindu*). The *ojas*, when become sufficiently conserved and potentiated, eventually turns into the most powerful and creative energies of all, the *Kundalini-shakti*.

Since the medical orthodoxy is unlikely to accept existence of yogic entities such as the *Kundalini-shakti* or the *prana* in a hurry, it is futile to argue over the need for celibacy, with allopathic physicians. Repression of the sexual energy is by no means recommended in yoga, since it is bound to create a backlash. A certain moderation in sexual indulgence however, is eminently desirable. When true Yoga unfolds in the form of the upwardly exerting *ojas*, the sexual drive is said to get channelled and sublimated to occasion immensely more pleasurable sensations thanks to the activated *Kundalini*. Incidentally, a sustained practice of yoga puts you in much greater control of your sexual urge, while giving you a much more energetic sex life.

P. Physical Asana

As already explained, too much emphasis on physical *asanas* is avoidable. A daily practice of three or four physical postures for five to ten minutes should suffice. A good combination can be one comprising one forward bending *asana* (e. g. *paschimottanasana*), one backward bending *asana* (e. g. *bhujangasana*) and one *asana* after principal meals (*vajrasana*). *Padmasana* may synergistically add to the efficacy of meditation. Here is a table of some useful *asanas:*

> प्रयत्नशैथिल्यानन्तसमापत्तिभ्याम्।
>
> ***Posture is mastered by leaving effort and identifying with the Infinite.***
>
> —*Yoga Sutra, Patanjali:* II, 47

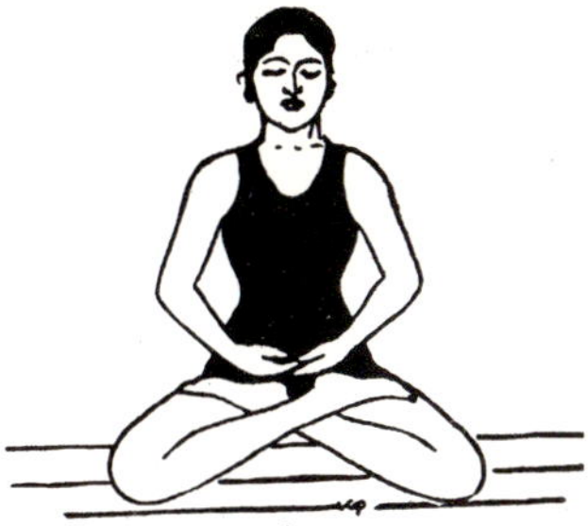

Padmasana

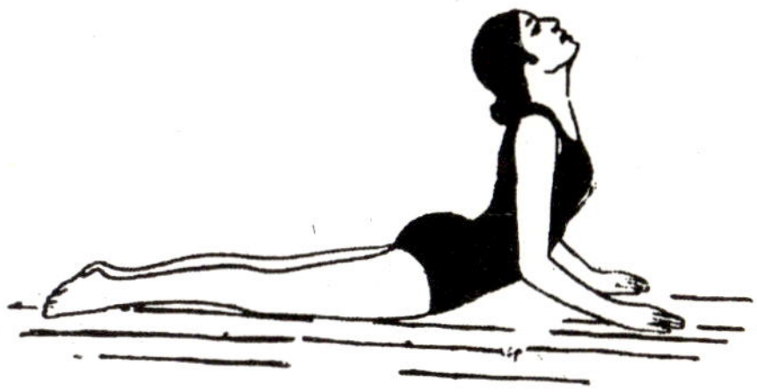

Bhujangasana

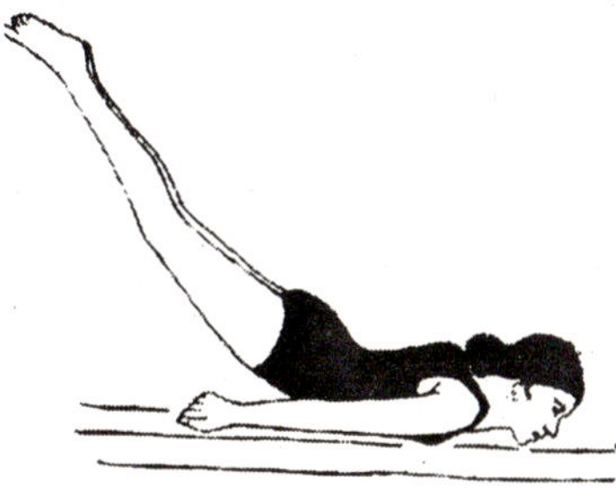

Shalabhasana

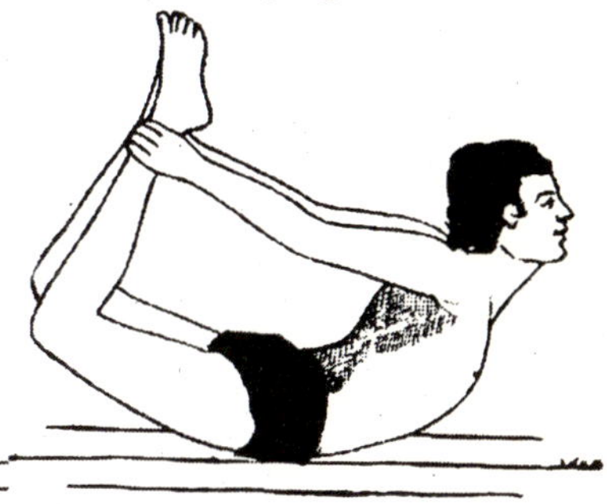

Dhanurasana

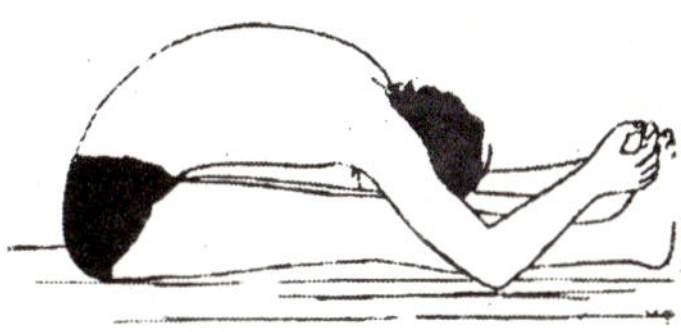

Paschimottanasana

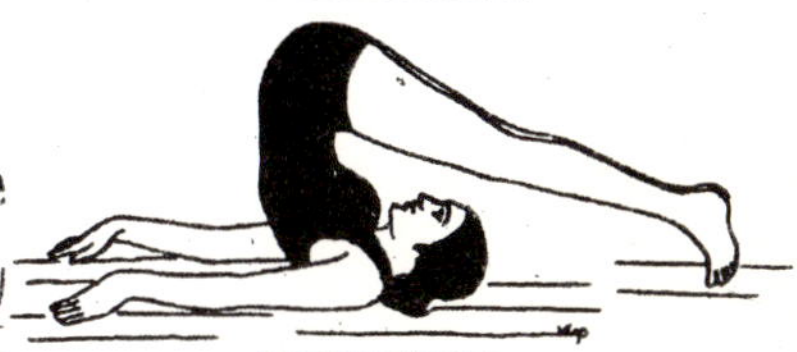

Halasana

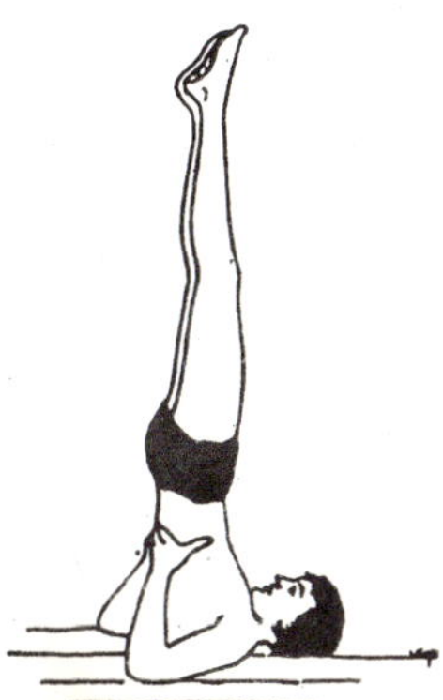

Sarvangasana

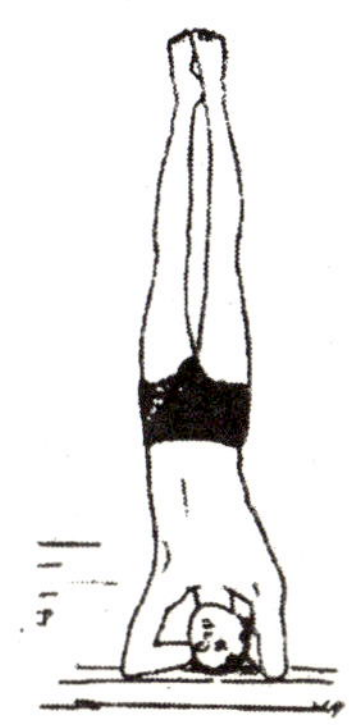

Shirsasana

Asana	Good for	Contra-indication
1. *Padmasana*	Meditation, Nervous system	Knee problem, Varicose veins
2. *Vajrasana*	Constipation, Hydrosil, Hernia, Sciatica	Bad ankle, Knee fracture
3. *Bhujangasana*	Waist-sprain, Arthritis, Sciatica, Diabetes, PMS, Respiratory troubles, Slip-disc, Sprained neck	Hernia, Hyperactive thyroid
4. *Shalabhasana*	Stomach, Sciatica, Heart	High blood pressure, Heart trouble, Peptic ulcer, Hernia, Intestinal trouble
5. *Dhanurasana*	Constipation, Obesity	High BP, Hernia, Duode nal/Peptic ulcer
6. *Pawan-muktasana*	Obesity, Gastric	Cervical spondylitis
7. *Sarvangasana*	Lungs, Neck, Digestive system, PMS, Brain	High BP/Low BP, Heart problem, Weak eye capillaries, Slip-disc, Spondylitis
8. *Paschimo-ttanasana*	Obesity, Gastric, Kidney trouble, Pancreas, Spine	Hernia, Enlarged liver or spleen, Sprained neck, High BP, Constipation, Slip disc
9. *Halasana*	Intestines, Kidneys, Pancreas, Diabetes, Obesity	Cervical spondylitis, Sciatica, Slip disc, Sprained neck
10. *Shirsasana*	Brain, Blood circulation	Weak eyes, High BP, Heart trouble
11. *Surya-namaskara*	Digestion, Blood circulation, Respiratory system, Physical growth of children	Back pain, Fever, Pregnancy, Slip disc, PMS

Q. Questioning

Just as true knowledge emerges from doubt, true faith has its origin in questioning. Yoga and meditation, in the ultimate analysis, are all about faith. No amount of yoga theory can conclusively prove yoga the way *a priory* facts such as 2+2 = 4 can be. Every yoga practitioner therefore, however much rationally inclined, must in the end, take a leap of faith when he turns to yoga. True faith however, as distinct from superstition, does not and should not come overnight. unless one is a seeker of the highest order. For faith, in order that it is strong enough to carry you through the enormous vicissitudes of life, must have the underpinnings of questioning. A good way to become mentally geared to yoga is by taking a break and asking yourself the basic questions. The great Muktananda was fond of jolting his prospective disciples out of their stupor like existence with a deceptively simple, almost casual enquiry, "*Where are you going*?" And coming from an enlightened yogi, the simple question sufficed to spark off a stream of yoga in many a visitor. The readiness to question oneself about the real purpose and manner of living must be supplemented by questioning the outer perceptions once you have set your mind on yoga. *Don't take the guru on face value, don't follow the yoga teacher, don't believe the astrologer, don't accept the hymns and mantras, don't go to the shrine, don't trust books—without first questioning them, if you are not to be misled.* Some of the questions have to be directed at 'the other'. For the most part however, this questioning has to go about inside enabling you to reach a definite conclusion, and withdraw if necessary without occasioning hostility. Care must be taken to ensure that even as you question, you are open to new learning and relatively free of bias.

R. Regularity

The virtue of being regular in yoga, like in any other pursuit, should hardly need any explaining. In yoga, the need to underline regularity arises largely in the context of *japa*—the most powerful form of yoga—although regularity in the matter of dietary habits, cold water bath and like other areas cannot be lost sight of. In *japa* meditation, try to be regular in the following respects:

(a) Whatever be the duration, choose a *fixed time* for meditating on your mantra or the hymn. Sunrise and sunset times are particularly conducive to meditation, since at these times the mind naturally has a tendency to be absorbed in itself. Best time for meditation is close to the *Brahma-muhurtha* between 4 a.m. and 6 a.m., firstly because it is spiritually the most rewarding and secondly, because it is likely to cause the least dislocation in your day long busy schedule.

(b) Like in choosing time, choose *a fixed place* for daily meditation; a place that gives you relative privacy and is less frequented by family members. As you meditate daily, the place itself becomes charged with spiritual energy making your *japa* more and more effortless.

(c) Do the *japa* either sitting in the lotus posture (*Padmasana*) or lying down in *shavasana. The true meaning of asana is any bodily posture that can hold your body still and your spine, straight for the inner energies to get properly channelled;* so don't read too much into the posture as a vehicle of meditation.

(d) Cut down the stimulations—close the doors and curtains, shut off all noise and music and if possible, wrap a handkerchief over your closed eyes. A degree of sense withdrawal or '*Pratyahara*' is necessary for meditation to gain in depth and effect.

(e) Use the same woollen or jute blanket—folded or spread depending on your *asana*—to insulate yourself from the ground when meditating and do not wash it very often. It prevents the vibrational energy gener-

> ated in the course of sustained meditation from getting dissipated . In due course the fabric itself becomes suffused with the energies so as to become a valuable aid to your daily meditation.

Again, do not despair if you find the regularity missing from your daily meditation initially. Regularity is a matter of degree that should not be too much insisted upon in the initial stages. *Any time of the day is fine for meditation as is any place.* Avoid long meditation however, just after a heavy meal.

S. Slowing Down

In a civilization that is all the time putting pressure on us subliminally to grab more and move ahead, the dividing line between happiness and pleasure has all but disappeared. Material acquisitions and consumption seem to be the only thing that our consumerist culture now would have us believe, are worth aspiring for. Yet the high incidence of suicides, mental breakdowns and life style diseases such as AIDS, cancer, strokes, depression and diabetes in the developed nations is proof enough that *happiness is not a commodity*. Modern psychologists have now conducted enough research to conclude that *people for whom affluence is the uppermost concern in life tend to suffer from abnormally high degree of stress, depression and a host of behavioural and physiological disorders*. No wonder D. H. Lawrence called money modern man's "*vast collective madness*". If you're the type who has 'everything in life but time for yourself', take a long pause and a fresh look at your life. Beyond the basic necessities of living, the good things of life are to be savoured in leisure and better still, shared with others. Workaholics who grind themselves in a 14 hour-a-day schedule in a maddening rush to become rich, successful and famous are unwittingly putting so much pressure on their own system that onset of psychological trauma and physical incapacitation becomes a matter of time. In our stressed-out world, the primitive fight-or-flight response that helped our ancestors survive, has taken the form of what has been called a "stew or chew" response. Chronically raised levels of stress hormones engender a vicious cycle in which stress occasions habitual shallow breathing that in turn generates more stress. Slow, rhythmic "belly breathing", as against the more common "chest breathing" is among the most potent and handy anti-stress medicines that we have. The average breathing rate (in and out) is about 15 cycles per minute. With mind-body techniques, it can be slowed down to below 10 cycles with great therapeutic benefits. *Researcher Alice D. Domar of Harvard Medical School has shown that deep diaphragmatic breathing can significantly combat depression, infertility and PMS related disorders.* Breathing—and breathing alone among human physiological responses—is both voluntary and involuntary. Which means that, conjoined with the emotional state, it can give rise to either a negative or a positive cycle. Breathing slower you unwind. More significantly, unwinding you breath slower.

Often I have found people say that they are all for yoga and meditation, but that they simply don't have the time. On such occasions one is able to do nothing but feel sorry for them. For they never cared to discover in the first place that 20 minutes of meditation each morning is capable of giving them such new levels of creative energy and efficiency that the work that earlier required 14 hours can be now completed more clinically in, may be, 6 hours flat! More importantly, it can cushion them against the probability of such rough handling by forces of nature as is likely to leave them with all the goodies, all the time in the world and no strength to enjoy them. My sincere advice to all the reasonably well off persons then, would be to go easy on fresh acquisitions, brace up for a leaner pay package if necessary and in return find more quality time for themselves that is used much more creatively in the silent practice of yoga. A good way of spending quality time with yourself is by serious reading of books like *'Autobiography of a Yogi'*, Muktananda's *'I Have Become Alive'*, *'Ramakrishna and his Disciples'* by Christopher Isherwood and K. N. Rao's *'Yogis, Destiny and the Wheel of Time'*. The beauty of these books is that they read like novels and teach like scriptures.

T. Travelling

Travelling has always been instinctively dear to man. In the Western cultures, travelling is largely looked forward to as the means to explore, while in the Indian tradition, it often takes the form of pilgrimage. The scriptures recommend as astrological remedy, visits to religions towns, hills and rivers that have the power to cleanse and energize astral bodies by working on your karma. Yet, people used to a degree of sophistication find the thronging crowds at the religious places of Varanasi, Tirupati, Vaishno Devi, Prayaga, Haridwar and Rameswaram a bit too much to handle. The next time you plan an excursion in India and are caught between a desire to explore nature and a wish to be at a pilgrim centre, try to combine both. There are any number of less frequented places in India that are of equal spiritual import and yet bring you face to face with the largely unspoilt charm of hills, jungles and rivers. The ritualistic sacrifice of animals that is unfortunately still prevalent at some of these places, especially the *shakti* centres, is best avoided without becoming judgemental or getting worked up over the presence or lack of religious sanction behind the offering. Some such places are suggested here, in the fond hope that the reader, specially the Westerner, would take the clue and find many more such places on his own:

Place	Nearest convenient Rly Station	Nearest Airport	Spiritual significance	Tourist attraction
1. Vindhyachal	Mirzapur	Varanasi	*Shakipitha*, Yogi Hans Baba's *Ashram*	Hills, Jungles
2. Naimish-aranya	Lucknow	Lucknow	Meditation ground of ancient seers	Thick forests
3. Vrindavana	Mathura	New Delhi	*Govardhana, Krishnabhumi*	Close to Taj Mahal, Agra
4. Kurukshetra	Kuruk-shetra	New Delhi	Site of *Mahabharata*, Holy pond	On Delhi—Kashmir route
5. Kedarnath	Dehradun	New Delhi	Shiva abode	The Himalayas
6. Girnar	Ahmeda-bad	Ahmedabad	Abode of Lord Dattatreya	Hills/Jungles
7. Amark-antaka	Bhopal	Bhopal	Ancient *Siddha* place	The Narmada, Scenic beauty
8. Jwaladevi/ Chamunda	Chandi-garh/ Pathankot	Chandi-garh	*Shaktipithas*	Kangra valley of Himachal Pradesh
9. Madhuban/ Chhinna-mastika	Dhanbad	Ranchi	Jain Pilgrim Centre/ *Shaktipitha*	Hills/Jungles, Falls

U. Uncork

It sounds empty philosophy, and in my weak moments, I am myself prone to be tentative. Trust me however; it is one of the most profound secrets of life that all the solutions to all your problems lie in your bosom waiting to be tapped. For, inside you breathes the dormant, yet all powerful self—not in the metaphysical sense, but as a concrete reality—composed of your dreams, talents, creativity, ambitions, and on the flip side, your insecurities, complexes and rivalries. The constructive part of your self stems from the potential 'you' that came into existence the moment you were born. The destructive part of your self on the other hand comprises the compulsions thrust upon us by our external setting in the shape of career blues, marital tensions, physical ailments and social conflicts. So long as we lead a worldly life, we have to meet worldly obligations, and this cannot be accomplished by becoming a recluse. On the other hand, too much fretting, running about and generally, 'living at the surface' only lets the hostile outside forces get the better of you by slowly cutting you off from your inner reservoirs of strength. If you would triumph over your external difficulties, then uncork your inner self you must. The same situation that looked gloomy, hopeless and scary, may arouse your inner capabilities to begin looking absorbing, stimulating and exciting. One sure-fire way to take the lid off is writing. *Researchers have found that people who wrote about traumatic events for 20 minutes-a-day thrice a week, had about half the number of doctor-visits as compared to people who did not write.*

If a scientific basis for this approach was still required, then have a look at what modern physicists and consciousness researchers have to say about the dynamics of human perception. Scientists are now discovering that our beliefs, thoughts, expectations and desires can decisively impact our biological core and redefine our cells, tissues and organs. Research is also showing that our perceptions are not exclusively or even predominantly the outcome of external stimuli, but are shaped in no small measure, by our anticipation of what will happen, by past experience and sundry other factors. Findings on the powerful placebo effect and the famous pseudo heart operations of 1950s are a pointer in this direction. All perception therefore, in significant measure, is 'Extrasensory Perception'.

V. Vegetarianism

The reason why I have chosen to discuss vegetarianism under a separate head, as distinguished from dietary advice in general, is that this is an aspect having important ethical and ecological ramifications quite aside from the more obvious medical concerns. Studies have confirmed that vegetarians as a group are healthier than the general population. Till the other day scientists thought that all the body needed to function optimally was carbohydrates, protein, fat, minerals, vitamins and water. Now they have discovered " life savers" in *phytochemicals(phyto* means plant) that abound in fruits and vegetables such as garlic(!), spinach, fenugreek, cabbage, oranges/lemons, grapes, tomatoes and papaya. *Meat is found to contain about 14 times the pesticide residue as plant food. Furthermore, compared to the meat eaters, white cells of vegetarians have been found to be twice as effective in destroying cancer cells.* When an animal is slaughtered for meat, its body profusely secretes certain neuro-excitatory hormones that are passed on to the flesh-eaters to occasion hypertension, gout, arthritis, neurological disorders, kidney malfunctioning and a host of other ailments. Vegetarianism in general is a big insurance against these diseases. Aside from the health considerations, the food cycle operates such that meat is by far the most resource guzzling, among the food options available to man, and thus militates against the yoga spirit of charity, sharing and co-existence. *While 25 gallons of water are required to produce one pound of wheat, 5000 gallons go into producing one pound of beef. Similarly, it needs 78 calories of fossil fuel to produce one calorie of beef, as against two calories of the same fuel for one calorie of soyabean.* With the rising world population outstripping our natural resources of land, water and forest, it is imperative that we reduce our meat-intake and gradually shun it altogether in order to avoid destruction of environment, and along with it, of mankind. Global warming, top soil erosion and deforestation may all be avoided in large measure if the world population takes to vegetarianism.

As regards the last but not the least of arguments against meat eating viz. , not to kill for hunt and pleasure, this surely is the most easily heard reason for staying vegetarian. Yet the issue is more tricky than it *prima facie* appears. Those who relish meat and have the intellectual brilliance to rationalize this, put forward the scientifically sound argument that since by definition, each bacteria, fungus, plant—verily each tissue and cell—is a living being, *we cannot conceivably eat and drink without necessarily killing.* To me however, it appears that human life was intended by the Supreme Intelligence to be largely an exercise in avoiding of extremes and taking the golden middle path for the most part, given the infirmities of the flesh. In '*Autobiography of a Yogi*' Yogananda's Guru, resurrected Christ-like after his physical death, tells the worthy disciple how astral beings, who are but the evolved version of mankind, need no food to nourish their '*bodies*' the way we do. So long as our Yeatsean sensibility is *"sick with desire and fastened to an animal it knows not"*, we are bound to kill life in some form or the other, as soon as we eat. But surely, in God's evolutionary scheme, the life of a bacteria or even that of a 'feeling' plant does not hold quite the same significance as that of an animal, or man himself. If the meat eaters' logic was taken to its conclusion, then they should have no compunction in going so far as to commit murder for human flesh, since in the end, 'it was all a matter of killing some or the other form of life'. The *karmic* law, I suspect, applies to us in such a way that we have to willy nilly play a snakes-and-ladders game. *We can neither totally avoid the snakes nor can be denied the ladders. The key to reaching the goal of life is in playing the game so astutely as to be repulsed by the smallest of snakes, and catapulted by the bigger among the ladders.* If we have to necessarily kill in order to survive, then we must kill life of the most elementary kind.

The desirability of a strictly vegetarian diet, as one would guess, assumes added significance in yoga, more so if the seeker opts for spiritual initiation or '*diksha*'. However, vegetarianism should not become a fetish for those who are otherwise keen on initiation with a degree of commitment. The beauty of *shaktipat-yoga* lies in its effortlessness, and *Siddha* Gurus never advise repression of instincts—urge for meat–eating being one of them—on the yoga path. K. N. Rao describes how his Guru allowed his initiated disciples (mostly Bengalis who have almost a biologically rooted liking for fish!) to have fish, to start with. My own Guru seldom shows his displeasure at his disciples eating meat, preferring to remain reticent on the issue and instead, urging them to become more intense and regular in *japa*. Underlying this approach is perhaps the knowledge of the Gurus that the effort wasted on the inner struggle to avoid eating meat pays much greater dividends, if it is instead, diverted towards concentrating on mantra repetition. Once the mantra starts taking roots, it starts changing everything about you from within including your food preferences. The disciples, post *diksha*, must therefore, try to curb meat eating gradually rather than wrestle with their 'non-vegetarian self' with full awareness that the *japa* would take care of the rest. Having said this, I must add that instructions post *diksha* differ from one Guru to another, and no general rules can be rigidly prescribed by outsiders in this matter of esoteric import.

W. Water Therapy

It is amusing how the commonest of things of everyday use hold some of the biggest secrets of yoga. Water certainly is one of them, as use of water in different forms(ice, water and steam), at different temperatures (hot ,cold and tepid) and from different processes (plain, magnetic or mineral) acts as a powerful instrument of yoga. Let us see how:

(a) Cold water

Readers would recall that *Shaucha* or internal cleanliness is one of the commandments (*Niyamas*) of *Patanjali-yoga*. The need for having a daily bath from the point of view of hygiene can hardly be overemphasized. Medical science can also be counted upon to favour cold rather than hot water for daily bath since it is gentler on the body and is said to improve blood circulation and aid moisture-retention. While the New Age medical science may go on discovering more and more merit in a daily cold water bath, its significance from the yoga point of view goes much beyond the physical. Somehow, frequent cold water baths seem to wash away the negative energies that threaten to envelope you in course of the fatigue, the tensions and the anxieties arising from the everyday routine, and temporarily give the feeling of a 'new birth'. It has been my experience that a cold water bath definitely improves your astral vibrations and turns you automatically in 'the yoga mood'—some thing that you can yourself notice over a short period of practice and introspection. So next time, when you are feeling low, angry or simply lethargic, just take a plunge into the pool or take to the shower, remembering only one thing—the water should be cold to very cold in summers and lukewarm to tolerably cold in the winters.

(b) Hot water

Take a bucketful of tolerably hot water with a good amount of common salt thrown in. Put your both legs in the hot water, sitting in your easy chair. Enjoy the warmth and the refreshing feel that quickly does away all the fatigue. Although most of us are aware of the relaxation that this simple chore brings, I decided to include this as part of water therapy only after I once found it sending waves of inner energy surging up my spine when I was least prepared for it.

(c) 'Mineral' water

Take a large enough copper vessel—a jug preferably—and

keep about two big glassfuls of clean water in it overnight, to be taken first thing in the morning. This 'mineral' water obtained free of cost with least exertion is among the simpler remedies to put your stomach back in order and improve your condition in many diseases. Drink 8 to 10 glasses of water—squeezing in half-a-lemon once or twice.

(d) *Jala-neti*

Many of the diseases in these times arise due to environmental and dietary pollution. One simple, yet powerfully yogic *kriya* that tones up the immune system and cleanses the internal passages is *Jala-neti*. Regular practice of *Jala-neti* is a very effective means of maintaining and promoting physical health by removing wastes and toxins and aiding free flow of *prana*. In *Jala-neti*, you take a kettle–like copper vessel of suitable design (available in the market) that has a nozzle protruding at one end. The vessel is then filled up with clean, tepid water that has some common salt dissolved in it. Then you tilt the vessel placing its nozzle next to your nostrils in such a way that the water is sucked in from one nostril, and through the nasal passage, oozes out from the other. Meanwhile, you have to breathe orally, using the nostrils only for *Jala-neti*. Care must be taken to ensure that all water ingested thus is sniffed out from the nostrils at the end by breathing out in bursts. Although *Jala-neti* is not believed to do any harm even if practised imperfectly by a novice, it is advisable to get in touch with a yoga teacher to get a demo before you get started.

X. X-Zone

One of the five constituents of *niyama* or restraint that the eight fold yoga teaches us is surrender in God's Will, or *Ishwara pranidhana*. After you have used all your ingenuity and foresight in planning the last details of your present and future, you still often live to regret the fact that things did not quite turn out the way they should have. Depression, loss of self-esteem, blurred reality perception, tense relationships are some of the after-effects of 'things getting out of hand'. A little dispassionate thinking would however, show that most of these complications arise from a basic ignorance of life's guiding influence. In the Yoga theory, the exact word for destiny is *adrshta* or the 'unseen'. It is here that the value of surrender to God's Will becomes evident. Beyond a point, the eagerness to see the unseen is not only pointless, but also counterproductive. The sooner we reconcile ourselves to the fact that there is a higher law operating, that overrides, and occasionally overturns our little laws of everyday living (very often in our own interest), the better it will be. Looking back I know it for a fact that some of the prayers I fervently made to God in the last few years, would have spelt doom for me had these been granted!

This unseen face or what I call, 'the X Zone' of life, instead of scaring us, must make us place greater trust in the inherent goodness of Nature and the Higher Existent. Yogananda once observed that God occasionally denies us our desired things only because He has better gifts in store for us. The imperfect mind and senses play many tricks on us and it is often the case that what we *need* is substantially different from what we *desire*. So the next time you are being torn by conflict and indecision in a particularly fluid situation and are unable on your own, to go this or that way, just leave the X Zone to take care of itself. When time is ripe and God's Will translated, you will be surprised to find that answers have come from almost nowhere, or at least from those unlikely corners of existence which could by no means be accessed earlier. So, do plan the 'p's and 'q's of your life to the best of your ability, but have respect for the X Zone which rightfully belongs to God, and is best left under His cares.

Y. Yoga-nidra

It is all very well for the advanced practitioners of yoga, specially meditation, to rave about their accomplishments, real or imagined. But the neophyte who needs 'to stand before he walks and walk before he runs', must really be nursed through an inevitable period of psychological uncertainty that separates a hedonistic mind-set from the yogic orientation. To most yoga beginners, the highly esoteric *Shaktipat-yoga*, at least early on, is likely to be elusive for reasons beyond their control. And a majority might find reciting the astrologically indicated hymns in chaste Sanskrit, beyond them in the first go. Indeed, quite a few find it difficult to sit or lie down for ten minutes when they first attempt meditation. The problems are compounded for the Westerner, save the fact that he perhaps carries a much stronger will. All these constraints, as I have explained earlier, can be overcome provided one perseveres and innovates. But this takes time, and the beginner must have some concrete external prop in the interregnum to start meditation and carry on. The best help that I have been able to think of in these circumstances is the *Yoga–nidra* practice. All one needs to practise *Yoga-nidra* is an audio cassette that dispenses a half-an-hour long taped instruction on sense–withdrawal (*Pratyahara*) technique that you scrupulously follow lying down comfortably, and that gradually ushers in a state of deep enough meditation. A good way to get started on Yoga is by buying the audio cassette, or preferably the CD, brought out by the *Bihar School of Yoga, Munger, India,* that is available in both, Hindi and English versions, and is perhaps recorded (I am not sure) in Swami Niranjanananda's impressive voice.

Yoga-nidra is a very simple practice in guided meditation that does not make any demands on the practitioner. You choose the privacy, silence and semi-darkness of your room, lie down in *shavasana*, and go on listening and mentally obeying the simple instructions. The crucial thing is not to fall asleep and to allow consciousness to effortlessly hover between the subconscious and the conscious; something that is conducive to deep relaxation, healing and higher awareness. The brain occasions *delta* waves in deep sleep, *alpha* waves in the relaxed state and alternating *alpha* and *beta/theta* waves in the *Yoga-nidra* state. The rapid onset of dense patterns of alpha waves interspersed with beta/theta waves is the key to the *Yoga-nidra* efficacy.

Brain Waves	**Frequency (Hz.)**	**Characteristic State**
Delta	0.5—4	Deep Sleep
Theta	4—7.5	Sleep, Drowsiness, Some Creativity
Alpha	7.5—13	Relaxation, Creativity, Peak Performance
Beta	13—40	Alertness, Arousal, Stress

Research shows that the stressed urban population now increasingly experiences in large measure, only the extreme *beta* and *delta* states in alternate bursts, nearly completely missing out on the soothing *alpha* and *theta* states that aid creativity, recharging and healing. Any internal or external aid that yields *theta* and specialy, the *alpha* waves, does wonders to man's ravaged psyche and physique.

Critics have often compared meditative states, specially *Yoga-nidra*, to hypnosis. However, the higher meditative states, of which *Yoga-nidra* is but a precursor, are qualitatively different from the hypnotic state inasmuch as advanced meditation engenders a vastly expanded 'superconsciousness' while hypnosis tends to seriously curtail consciousness. In the meditative state, just as in hypnosis, sensory inputs that are ordinarily supplied to the brain through *ida* and *pingala*, doubtless reduce or dry up altogether. But unlike in hypnosis, the ordinarily closed central sensory channel of the *susumna* gets partially or completely opened up in meditation giving the practitioner a kind of sensory awareness that is livelier and expanded many times over, and is marked by greatly healing 'extra sensory perceptions'. Not surprisingly, scientists in breakthrough lab-studies on the physical correlates of yoga states, have come across confounding brain wave-patterns that do not fit any label. Since these waves do not conform to any of the three normal states, sleep, dream and wakefulness, researchers are now inclined to favour this as the take-off point for closer scrutiny of the mystical "fourth state".

The psycho-physical benefits of *Yoga-nidra* practice are considerable and many. In the least, it gives the yoga beginner a launching pad for meditation. However, the *Yoga-nidra* practitioner, over a period, must try and graduate from a dependence on *Yoga-nidra* to more spiritual meditative practices comprising silent repetition of 'Om' or Sanskrit hymns, and culminating in *Shaktipat* meditation. This is not unlike the case of a feeble legged person using a walking stick to begin with, only to discard it once his limbs have become sturdy enough. A good way to be on track is to make a subconscious resolve in the powerfully receptive *sankalpa* stage of *Yoga-nidra*, such as this: "I shall go far and deep in spiritual meditation". *Yoga-nidra* is very efficacious in hypertension, cardiac problems, neurosis, insomnia and several other psychosomatic illnesses. It should, however be avoided by those suffering from epilepsy or psychotic depression.

Z. Zeroing-in

Science and the Church are no longer strangers. Increasingly it transpires that Darwin seriously erred in putting man and animal on the same continuum; that man is after all created in God's 'Own Image'. No matter how many billions of our species crowd the globe, no matter how many haves steep themselves in beastly obsession with *nidra, ahara* and *maithuna* (sleep, sausage and sex), and no matter how many have-nots subsist as mere extensions of the belly; there would always be room for the equipped and the discerning among us to rise above all limitations and touch the skies. Perhaps the underprivileged can be excused for the present, from exploring higher realms. For their *karmic* dictates appear to be such as to permit more purposeful living only in subsequent incarnations. But there can really be no justification for the more endowed among us to let our divine potential go waste. Each of us must, through Yoga, gain control over events in some measure, rather than be overtaken by them. The *chakras*, the *prana*, the *siddhis* and the *kundalini-shakti* are for real; we only need to determinedly uncover them and harness the tremendous higher energies in one-pointedness for Nature to ignite and do our bidding. This zeroing-in on the Source with all our physical, mental and spiritual might, regardless of the initial trepidation and surrounding distractions, is the secret of Yoga. Disease, destruction and drift that today beset mankind, both in the developed West and the deprived East are in the end analysis, symptoms of our shallow, fragmented and dissipated living. From this we have to break open individually, before collectively.

To Recap

A. Seek astrological advice.
B. Digest *Bhagavad Gita.*
C. Cultivate charity as a habit.
D. Right diet is basic to yoga.
E. Work at down-sizing the ego.
F. Fast judiciously.
G. Be cautious in 'choosing' a guru.
H. Find out your humour type for greater self-awareness.
I. Introspect always.
J. Do *japa* silently, lovingly and with concentration.
K. Remember the karma concept as key to yoga.
L. Laughter does cure.
M. Music also does.
N. Nature care is best care.
O. Conserve *ojas.*
P. Be sensible about physical *asanas.*
Q. Question everything before you believe.

R. Be regular in diet and meditation.
S. Slow down, if the need be, to avoid being an early burn-out.
T. Combine love for nature and spiritual gains in excursion trips.
U. Uncork your latent complexes/energies for meeting the challenges.
V. Vegetarianism is desirable medically, ethically and ecologically.
W. Water can be used in many ingenious ways to heal.
X. After you have planned your future every bit, entrust the imponderables to God.
Y. Practice *Yoga-nidra* preparatory to more esoteric yoga practices.
Z. Human life is never without a purpose; find that out and zero-in for fulfillment.

Glossary

ADESHA (*ādeśa*): The "God–Commandment" received by a perfected yogi through his open crown centre, guiding his 'worldly' activities post Realization.

ADITYA HRDAYA STOTRA (*Āditya Hṛdaya Stōtra*): A Sanskrit hymn to the Sun God culled from the *Vālmiki Rāmāyaṇa* that is often prescribed as an effective astrological remedy for an afflicted Sun in one's natal horoscope.

ADRSHTA (*adṛṣṭa*): The "unseen" forces of destiny.

AHAṂKARA (*ahaṃkāra*): The *māyā*-induced feeling of 'I-ness' among mortals.

AHARA (*āhāra*): The "diet" that sustains the physical body; also implies meditation as nourishment for the subtle bodies.

AHIMSA (*ahiṃsā*): The observance of "non-injury": one of the five moral observances *(yama)* in Patanjali yoga, other four being *satya, asteya, brahmacharya* and *aparigṛaha.*

APANA (*apāna*): The "down-breath" or the expelling current of life energy instrumental in evacuating waste matter from the body.

ASANA (*āsana*): Any steady and relaxed "posture" that can hold the spine erect and facilitate upward thrusts of the rising *Kuṇḍalini*-energy.

ASHRAM (*āśram*): A hermitage where an adept normally resides in order to instruct and bless disciples. Also, a stage of life in the Hindu social order – the four stages in ascending chronological order being *brahmacharya* (brahmic pursuit), *gṛihasthya* (householder's), *vānaprastha* (forest-dwelling) and *sanyāsa* (renunciation).

ASHTANGA (*aṣṭāṅga*): The "eight–limbed" yoga enunciated by Patanjali comprising *yama, niyama, āsana, prāṇāyāma, pratyāhāra, dhāraṇā, dhyāna* and *samādhi.*

AYURVEDA (*āyurveda*): The Vedic "science of life" that is the native Indian system of medicine first mentioned in the Atharva Veda and later on detailed in the *Charaka Saṁhitā*.

BHAGAVAD GITA (*Bhagavat Gītā*): "Song of the Lord" that comes in the form of an episode in the *Mahābhārata,* and is the most inspiring of all Yoga scriptures.

BHAKTI YOGA (*bhakti yoga*): The yoga of "devotion" geared toward union with God through His continuous remembrance.

BHARATA (*Bharata*): The younger brother of Lord Rama who refused to ascend the Throne during the exile of Rama and ruled over the kingdom only as Rama's representative.

BHAVATITA DHYANA (*bhāvātīta dhyāna*): The Hindi equivalent of Transcendental Meditation (TM) that was popularised in the West by the likes of Mahesh Yogi.

BHUJANGASANA (*bhujaṇgāsana*): The backward bending "cobra posture" practised lying belly down.

BIJA MANTRA (*bīja mantra*): The monosyllabic and meaningless "seed mantra" generally associated with Tantricism and the seven chakras.

BRAHMA MUHURTHA (*Brahma muhūrtha*): The "brahmic hour" or time just before sun-rise that is most conducive to meditation.

CHAITANYA MANTRA (*chāitanya mantra*): A "conscious" mantra charged with the living force of a Realized yogi that is the most powerful aid to meditation.

CHAKRAS (*chakras*): The psycho-energetic vortices or "wheels" that are often depicted as "lotuses" and refer to the hierarchic junction points of astral nerve tubes that can be roughly identified with the nerve plexuses of the physical body. The seven chakras are the *mūlādhāra, svādhiṣṭhāna, maṇipura, anāhata, visuddha, ājnā,* and *sahasrāra.*

CHAPATIS (*chapātīs*): A type of bread made of wheat flour, and part of the staple north Indian diet.

CHITTA (*chitta*): One of the key concepts in Patanjali-yoga that is roughly the equivalent of mind or finite consciousness.

DARSHANA (*darśana*): The auspicious and healing "sight" of an exalted yogi.

DESI GHEE (*desī ghee*): Clarified butter, mostly consumed in India and often used in *Āyurveda* to go with medicines.

DHANURASANA (*dhanurāsana*): The backward bending "bow posture" practised lying belly down.

DHYANA (*dhyāna*): The stage of "contemplation" in Patanjali–yoga, preparatory to the ultimate state of Samādhi.

DIKSHA (*dīkṣhā*): Spiritual initiation of a disciple by a perfected yogi, usually with the aid of a mantra.

DOSHA(S) (*dōṣa*): The bodily humours (*tridōṣas*)—*vāta, kapha* and *pitta*–recognized in *Āyurveda* as the key to the individual state of health or disease.

DVIJA (*dvija*): The "twice born" or the mantra-initiated; *dīkṣhā* being viewed as the second birth.

EKAGRATA (*ekāgratā*): "One pointedness" of attention that is conducive to yoga.

GAYATRI (*Gāyatrī*): One of the most important Sanskrit mantras invoking the Universal Consciousness. Systematic and faithful recital of the *Gāyatrī* is both, a potent astrological remedy and a valuable support in meditation.

GHATANA (*ghatanā*): "Mitigation" of suffering that is said to result from a serious practice of Yoga.

GHERANDA-SAMHITA (*Gheraṇḍa-Saṃhitā*): A classic medieval text on hatha yoga attributed to sage *Gheraṇḍa.* Comprising 351 stanzas in seven chapters, it forms the basis of much of contemporary yoga.

GRAHA SHANTI (*gṛaha śānti*): "Propitiation of planets" that mitigates astrologically indicated afflictions in one's natal chart and the consequent suffering.

GUNA(S) (*guṇa*): The principal "strands" or constituents of nature – *sattva* (light), *rajas* (activity) and *tamas* (sloth) – that among other things, interact and give rise to man's disposition.

GURU (*Guru*): The self-realized master-teacher who, "dispels darkness" and is the "weighty one," transmitting the supreme Grace to a deserving disciple, and guiding him on the yoga path.

GURU PURNIMA (*Guru Pūrṇimā*): The festive and auspicious occasion of celebrations in honour of the Guru that comes every July on the full moon.

HALASANA (*halāsana*): The forward bending "plough posture" practised upside down.

HANS (*haṃs*): The "swan" or the soul.

HATHA-YOGA (*haṭha-yoga*): A yogic discipline of "forceful yoga" geared toward reaching the Yoga state of *Kuṇḍalini* awakening and Self–realization by means of perfecting the body.

HATHA-YOGA-PRADIPIKA (*Haṭha-Yoga-Pradīpikā*): The most acclaimed haṭha yoga scripture of medieval origin that seeks to reconcile the physical yoga with higher spiritual pursuits of *rāja yoga.* Comprising 389 couplets in four chapters, the text describes key techniques including postures, breath retention, seals (*mudrā*) and locks (*bandha*).

ISHVAR PRANIDHANA (*Īśhvar praṇidhāna*): The most important among the constituents of internal observances *(niyama)*, others being *shaucha, saṃtosha, tapas* and *svādhyāya*.

JADA MANTRA (*jaḍa mantra*): The "inert" mantra, usually obtained from books or an ordinary teacher.

JAPA (*japa)*: Silent and loving repetition of a sacred hymn or mantra that is the chief aid in meditation, capable of ushering in the Realized state.

KARA (*karā*): A metallic armlet often worn as an astrological remedy.

KARMA (*karma*): Physical, verbal or mental "action". Karma that is destined to be played out in the current life is *prārabdha*, that which is 'bound' to be played in future lives is *saṃchita karma*; that which is being created in the present life-time is *kṛiyāmāṇa karma.*

KARMA YOGA (*karma yoga*): The yoga of "detached action" in which one undertakes actions as an offering without anxiety for the fruits of these actions.

KAIVALYA (*kāivalya*): The ultimate state of isoloation in Patanjali Yoga in which liberation or complete transcendence of the narrow self occurs.

KATANA (*katanā*): "Elimination" of suffering that is said to result from a serious practice of Yoga.

KEVALA KUMBHAKA (*kēvala kumbhaka)*: A form of breath retention without inhalation and exhalation, and a key element in *prāṇāyāma* designed to facilitate Realization.

KOSHA (*kōṣa*): The "sheath(s)" that envelops the Consciousness starting from the coarsest – the physical body— ending up with the subtlest that comprises the Spirit itself.

KRIYA (*kṛiyā*): Involuntary movement(s) of the limbs following arousal of the *Kuṇḍalini*-energy that has a purifying physiological, psychological and spiritual effect.

KRIYA YOGA (*kṛiyā yoga*): The yoga of transmutative "action" that finds mention in scriptures including the *Bhagavad Gītā* and that was made popular in the West by Paramahansa Yogananda.

KUNDALINI (*kuṇḍalini*): The supreme energy that among humans, lies "coiled" and dormant at the spinal base. Through various yogic practices, it is capable of being awakened – surging up the central channel of susumna and piercing the seven *chakras* in succession, until it grants Enlightenment.

KUNDALINI YOGA (*kuṇḍalini yoga*): The type of yoga that seeks consummation through a systematic awakening of the *Kuṇḍalini*-energy.

LAYA YOGA (*laya yoga*): The yoga of "absorption" that seeks to dissolve the finite mind into the Infinite through contemplation and meditative practices.

MACHAN (*machān*): A raised wooden platform which a yogi in the Patanjali tradition often uses to seat himself and bless devotees.

MALA (*mālā*): A "rosary" often used as an aid to mantra repetition and meditation.

MANTRA YOGA (*mantra yoga*): The yoga comprising contemplative repetition *(japa)* of various mantras made up of certain fixed Sanskrit sounds.

MARKANDEYA PURANA (*Mārkaṇḍeya Purāṇa*): One of the earliest Purāṇic texts dating back to around third century BC and dealing specifically with yoga.

MOKSHA (*mokṣha*): The Hindu concept of liberation from the cycle of birth and death.

NADA (*nāda*): The subtle cosmic sound that underlies all Creation.

NADIS (*nāḍis*): The psycho-energetic nerve tubes or "conduits" that carry the life force *(prāṇa)* throughout the body. The three principal *nāḍis* are the *idā,* the *pingalā* and the *susumnā.*

NASIKAGRA (*nāsikāgra*): The "nose-tip" which actually implies the nose–root near the eyebrow–middle.

NIRVANA (*nirvāṇa*): An essentially Buddhist concept of enlightenment through "extinction" of all desires that however, has been hinted at in the Bhagavad Gita.

OM OR AUM (*Ōṃ*): The sacred, monosyllabic mantra symbolizing the Absolute. Next to the 'conscious' *mantra*, this and/or the *Gāyatrī*, can be the most powerful vehicle of yoga. 'Oṃ' as the symbol of the Absolute, is not exclusive to Hinduism. In Islam, its variant occurs as 'Amin'; in Christianity, as 'Amen'.

PADMASANA (*padmāsana*): The cross-legged "lotus" posture that helps the yoga practitioner sit comfortably for long and meditate with an erect spine, facilitating ascent of the *Kuṇḍalini*-energy.

PAPA (*pāpa*): Negative karma that leads to future suffering and bondage.

PARAKAYA PRAVESHA (*parakāyā pravesha*): The mysterious yogic technique of "entering another body" that is a key paranormal accomplishment known to all advanced yogis.

PARAMAHANSA (*paramahaṇsa*): The liberated yogi or the "supreme swan".

PARAVANI (*parāvāni*): The subtlest and most "transcendental speech" pattern, usually associated with perfected yogis. The other coarser modes of speech, in ascending order of differentiation, are *paśyanti, madhyamā* and *vaikhāri.*

PASCHIMOTTANASANA (*paschimottanāsana*): The forward bending "back extension posture" practised sitting down, legs unbending and extended.

PAWANAMUKTASANA (*pawanamuktāsana*): The "wind freeing" posture practised sitting down, legs extended.

PRANA (*prāṇa*): The life–sustaining force of the individual body and Cosmic Existence, akin to the Greek *pneuma* and the Latin *spiritus.*

PRANAYAMA (*prāṇāyāma*): A yogic technique of "breath control" designed to increase vital energy and effect steadiness of mind. Also, the fourth component of Patanjali's eight-fold yoga.

PRASADA (*prasāda*): The "grace" of a yogi that may come to the supplicants in many forms including eatables.

PRASAMKHYANA (*prasamkhyāna*): The state of "elevation" or ecstacy leading to discernment and the burning off of past karmas.

PUNYA (*punya*): Good karma that leads to future enjoyments and reduced suffering.

PURAKA (*pūraka*): The "inhalation" stage of *prānāyāma* signifying the inward flow of life energy (*prāṇa*) that fills all astral nerve tubes (*nāḍis*).

RAJASIKA (*rājasika*): One of the three *gunas* or dispositions that causes unrest and activity in humans.

RAJA YOGA (*rāja yoga*): Also known as the *aṣṭāṅga* or eight-limbed yoga, this "royal yoga" has its genesis in sage Patanjali's *Yoga – Sutra.* It comprises higher spiritual practices taking off from the preparatory discipline of haṭha–yoga.

RAMA RAKSHA STOTRA (*Rāma Rakṣhā Stōtra*): A Sanskrit hymn in the praise of Lord Rama that is often prescribed as a universal astrological remedy for all planetary afflictions in one's natal horoscope.

RECHAKA (*rechaka*): The "exhalation" stage of *prāṇāyāma* that signifies the outward flow of the life force.

RUDRA GRANTHI (*Rudra-granthi*): One of the three "knots" located at the *ājnā chakra*, blocking the free flow of the life force through the central channel of *susumnā*. The other two *granthis* are the *Brahma-granthi* located at the *mūlādhara*, and *Vishnu-granthi*, located at the heart centre.

SADHAKA (*sādhaka*): The serious yoga–practitioner who is granted paranormal experiences (*siddhis*) in the course of his efforts, but who is really after Enlightenment.

SAMADHI (*samādhi*): The "ecstatic" state of union with the

Absolute, realizable through meditation. Also, the eighth and final stage of Patanjali yoga. The Hindu tradition distinguishes between *savikalpa samādhi* in which traces of duality still remain, and *nirvikalpa samādhi* that signifies complete and permanent merger of the self in the Absolute.

SANKALPA (*saṅkalpa*): A "resolve" made at a most crucial, subconscious stage of *yoga–nidrā* that is said to take roots quickly and is greatly fulfilling.

SANYASA (*saṃnyāsa*): Avowed "renunciation" that refers to the fourth and final stage of life in the Vedas in which, having fulfilled one's worldly obligations, one is expected to pursue Realization.

SARVANGASANA (*sarvāṅgāsana*): The inverted "all limbs posture" practised with shoulder-stand.

SATTVIKA (*sāttvika*): The purest of the three *gunas* that causes peace and brightness in humans.

SHABDA (*śabda*): The lettered, meaningless or meaningful "sound" that occurs in the chain of evolution by which the primordial vibration *(spanda)* is made manifest.

SHAKTI (*śakti*): The divine cosmic energy that, according to Shaivite philosophy, is the feminine and dynamic aspect of the Absolute.

SHAKTIPAT (*śaktipāt*): The "descent of (spiritual) energy" from a perfected yogi that triggers the onset of yoga in the devotee.

SHALABHASANA (*śalabhāsana*): The back-bending "locust posture" practised lying belly down.

SHAMBHAVI MUDRA (*Śāmbhavi mudrā*): The most important "seal" in *haṭha yoga* and *Tantra* signifying a fixed, inward gaze with open pupils.

SHATKARMA (*śaṭkarma*): The "six (cleansing) acts" of *Gheraṇḍa- Saṃhitā* comprising a) *dhauti* (cleansing), b) *vasti* (enema), c) *neti*, d) *nauli*, e) *trātaka* (steady conscious gazing) and f) *kapāla bhāti* (skull lustre).

SHAVASANA (*śavāsana*): The relaxed "corpse posture" practised lying belly up. This is recommended as a follow up after practising each major *āsana.*

SHIRSHASANA (*śīrṣāsana*): The inverted "head posture" practised, legs extended and joined together with head-stand.

SHIVA-SAMHITA (*Śiva-Saṁhitā*): An important medieval text on haṭha yoga that is more conspicuous for containing a discourse between God (*Īśhwara*) and the Goddess (*Devī*).

SHODHANA (*shōdhana*): "Cleansing" that follows six purifying acts or the *satkarmas.*

SIDDHA (*siddha*): A fully illumined yogi who has "accomplished" God–perfection.

SIDDHA YOGA (*Siddha yoga*): The type of *Śaktipat yoga* (yoga of inner awakening by the Grace of a Siddha Guru) practised in the Muktananda tradition.

SIDDHI (*siddhi):* Paranormal "accomplishment(s)" that come in the course of yoga–pursuit (*sādhanā*). According to the *Yoga – Bhāṣya*, these are *animān (*miniaturization), *mahimān* (magnification), *laghimān* (levitation), *prāpti* (extension), *prākamya* (irresistible will), *vashitva* (mastery), *ishitritva* (lordship) and *kāma-avasyitva* (unfailing fulfillment of desires).

SURYA NAMASKARA (*sūrya namaskāra*): A set of twelve dynamic postures, best practised bathing the soft morning sun-light in "obeisance to the sun".

TAMASIKA (*tāmasika*): One of the three *gunas* or disposition that causes dullness and negativity in humans.

UPANISHADS (*Upaniṣads*): Ancient Hindu scriptures containing metaphysical speculations and seeds of Yoga. Also known as the *Vedānta* ("end of knowledge"), the Upanishads, together with the Vedas, form the cornerstone of Hinduism.

UTHANA (*uthanā*): "Rising above" suffering that is said to

result from a serious practice of Yoga.

VAJRASANA (*vajrāsana*): The "adamantine posture" practised sitting down with thighs tightened and legs close to the anus, supporting the buttocks. One of the few asanas that can be practised safely and profitably after a heavy meal.

VAK SIDDHI (*vāk siddhi*): The "perfect (infallible) utterance" that is the prerogative of a God-illumined yogi.

VAMA MARGA (*Vāma mārga)*: The radical "left hand path" of yoga emphasizing the infamous five m's (*pancha–ma–kāra*) as the route to Enlightenment.

VEDA(S) (*Veda*): The fountain-head of Hindu "knowledge" that comes in the form of four principal ancient scriptures – *Rig Veda, Atharva Veda, Sāma Veda* and *Yajur Veda.*

VIBHUTI (*vibhūti*): Psychic or paranormal powers that are conferred on the seeker in course of yoga-practice.

VISHNU (*Viṣṇu*): The chief Hindu Deity Who stands, in the Trinity, for the principle of preservation while Brahma signifies creation and Shiva, destruction. Rama, Krishna and Buddha are believed to be the more recent among the ten Vishnu incarnations (*dasāvatāra*).

VRTTI (*vṛtti*): "Fluctuations" of finite consciousness that, when restrained (*nirōdha*) by means of *yogic* practices, leads to ecstasy.

YOGA (*yoga*): The state of "union" with the Self realizable through various means.

YOGA NIDRA (*yoga nidrā*): A yogic state of sense-withdrawal hovering between sleep and wakefulness, that is claimed by some modern yoga-teachers to be greatly healing.

YOGA SUTRA (*Yoga Sūtra*): The classical medieval yoga text attributed to sage Patanjali.

Bibliography

1. *The Upanishads*—F. Max Mueller—Motilal Banarsidass, New Delhi.
2. *Vedic Hymns*—F. Max Mueller—Motilal Banarsidass, New Delhi.
3. *Shambhala Encyclopaedia of Yoga*—Georg Feuerstein, Ph.d.—Shambhala Publications, Boston.
4. *Spontaneous Healing* –Andrew Weil, M.D.—The Ballantine Publishing Group, New York.
5. *Where Are You Going* - Swami Muktananda—SYDA Foundation, New York.
6. *Light on the Path* - Swami Muktananda—SYDA Foundation, New York.
7. *Autobiography of a Yogi*—Yogananda Paramahansa –Los Angeles: Self –Realization Fellowship , 1998
8. *Yogis, Destiny and the Wheel of Time*— K.N. Rao—Vani Graphics, Lucknow.
9. *Yoga Systems of Patanjali*—J. H. Woods—Motilal Banarsidass, New Delhi.
10. *Yoga and Western Psychology*—G.C. Coster—Motilal Banarsidass, New Delhi.
11. *Life After Death*—Erica Simon—Sahni Publications, Delhi.
12. *Herbs That Heal*—H.K. Bakhru—Orient Paperbacks, Delhi.
13. *Reiki—108 Questions & Answers*—Paula Horan—Full Circle.
14. *Kundalini -A Modern View*—Darriel Irving—Jaico Publishing House
15. *Kundalini—The Secret of Life* - Swami Muktananda—SYDA Foundation, New York.

Index

NEW AGE BOOKS

THE ART AND SCIENCE OF PSYCHIC HEALING—*Larry M. McDaniel* and *Phyllis G. McDaniel*

Have you ever felt that there was more out there for you, if only you could obtain it. Have you ever wanted guidance, but didn't know where to go? Do you want to improve your financial picture and lifestyle? Do you seek a better and more fulfilling relationship, or a stronger marriage!.... If so, then this book is for you.

ISBN: 81-7822-030-x

BREATHE FREE—*Daniel Gagnon* and *Amadea Morningstar*

For the first time a self help book that tells it all. An expose on respiratory diseases and their natural treatment. Throughout you can to heal and manage: Common Cold, Earache, Allergies, Pleurisy, Cough, Bronchitis and Aids and Related Respiration Infection.

ISBN: 81-7822-018-0

CHAKRA ENERGY MASSAGE—*Marianne Uhl*

This book guides you into the fascinating world of the energy body. Drawing on the knowledge gained by Foot Reflexology Massage, it introduces you to the Chakra Energy Massage. She provides detailed information on the healing effects of gemstones and the powers of fragrant essences, as well as the vibrations of primal tones and various colours, all of which can be employed to effectively enhance your work with the Chakras.

ISBN: 81-7822-004-0

ENERGETIC HEALING—*Arnie Lade*

Embracing the Life Force is a guide to the inner landscape of subtle energy. In this groundbreaking book the role, manifestation, utility and healing power of our life force/energy is explored in a concise and informative fashion.

ISBN: 81-7822-005-9

FENG SHUI YOUR BODY—*Daniel Santos*

This breakthrough book applies the principles of Feng Shui, the ancient Chinese art of energy flow, to the most intimate house we inhabit—the human body. Postures, simple exercises, and innovative meditations, as well as a fascinating story of personal discovery, offer fresh insights into body-mind healing.

ISBN: 81-7822-012-1

35 GOLDEN KEYS TO WHO YOU ARE AND WHY YOU'RE HERE —*Linda C. Anderson*

Who am I? Why am I here? We ask ourselves these questions all the time. The answers determine our purpose in life, often our very survival. Here—for the very first time ever—are thirty-five golden keys to help you unlock the answers to these questions for yourself.

ISBN: 81-7822-037-7

HOW TO MASTER CHANGE IN YOUR LIFE: Sixty-Seven Ways to Handle Life's Toughest Moments—*Mary Carroll Moore*

This book offers sixty-seven powerful techniques to embrace each challenge with courage, love, and grace. It shows you how to not only cope with change but master it. You can actually use change to achieve personal goals and make your life more spiritually fulfilling.

ISBN: 81-7822-036-9

MAGNETIC HEALING—*Buryl Payne*

Discover the positive benefits of magnetism for improving your health and well being.

- ❑ What ailments can be treated with magnets?
- ❑ How do magnets work to heal the body?
- ❑ What is the correct way to use magnets?

Find the answers to these questions and more!

ISBN: 81-7822-002-4

PENDULUM HEALING HANDBOOK—*Walter Lubeck*

If you want to learn every aspect of how to use a pendulum, particularly in relation to methods of alternative healing, this book is for you. It answers the questions that normally occur following a person's first experiences with the pendulum.

ISBN: 81-7822-003-2

QUANTUM-TOUCH THE POWER TO HEAL—*Richard Gordon*

Quantum-Touch represents a major breakthrough in the art of hands-on healing. Whether you are a complete novice, a professional chiropractor, physical therapist, body worker, healer, or other health professional, Quantum-Touch allows you a dimension of power in your work that heretofore has not seemed possible. Since the body already knows how to heal itself, the practitioner need only apply the energy to affected areas.

ISBN: 81-7822-009-1

STRESS-FREE WORK WITH YOGA AND AYURVEDA—*Vinod Verma*

Dr. Verma's advice for a stress-free work environment begins with a daily yoga program—easy exercises that take a total of sixteen minutes a day! She shows you how to recognize the three basic Ayurvedic types so you can "read" the people you work with.

ISBN: 81-7822-000-8

UNCONDITIONAL BLISS—*Howard Raphael Cushnir*

This book is not about getting what you want. It's about allowing yourself to FEEL the way you want by embracing life one precious moment at a time...starting right now!

ISBN: 81-7822-013-x